Transcatheter Paravalvular Leak Closure

Grzegorz Smolka • Wojciech Wojakowski
Michal Tendera

Editors

Transcatheter Paravalvular Leak Closure

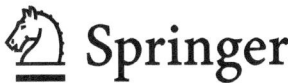 Springer

Editors
Grzegorz Smolka
Department of Cardiology and Structural
  Heart Diseases
Medical University of Silesia
Katowice, Poland

Wojciech Wojakowski
Department of Cardiology and Structural
  Heart Diseases
Medical University of Silesia
Katowice, Poland

Michal Tendera
Department of Cardiology and Structural
  Heart Diseases
Medical University of Silesia
Katowice, Poland

ISBN 978-981-10-5399-3   ISBN 978-981-10-5400-6   (eBook)
DOI 10.1007/978-981-10-5400-6

Library of Congress Control Number: 2017950005

Printed on acid-free paper

This Springer imprint is published by Springer Nature
The registered company is Springer Nature Singapore Pte Ltd.
The registered company address is: 152 Beach Road, #21-01/04 Gateway East, Singapore 189721, Singapore

Preface

Aortic stenosis and mitral regurgitation have become the most prevalent forms of valvular heart disease. They commonly require surgical interventions, including valve replacement. Although clinically significant postoperative paravalvular leaks are rather uncommon, they are recognized as an important clinical problem that may cause severe heart failure and intractable hemolysis.

In these patients, surgical reintervention is generally related to high perioperative risk. Therefore, transcatheter paravalvular leak treatment has attracted a lot of attention since its introduction in 2011.

Since then, transcatheter interventions have followed a difficult but successful path of development. The difficulties have been mostly linked to the technical issues, such as visualization of the defect, suboptimal delivery systems, and the lack of dedicated occluders. The success comes with the finding that the new method is feasible, clinically beneficial, and placing the patient at a lower risk than a repeated surgical procedure.

This book has been written to bring together most relevant data on the technical and clinical aspects of transcatheter paravalvular leak treatment and to point out to its limitations and future development.

The book should be of interest not only to interventional cardiologists focused on structural heart disease but also to general cardiologists, who often encounter patients with this problem in their clinical practice.

We are fortunate to have several leading experts in the field as authors. We would like to express our sincere thanks for sharing their expertise.

The book first covers surgical aspects of paravalvular leaks, indispensable in understanding of the problem, both in anatomical and clinical terms. Factors influencing the odds of PVL development, as well as surgical treatment options, are described.

Several chapters address the use of the available imaging techniques, such as different echo modalities, computed tomography and cardiac nuclear resonance in diagnosing PVL and its quantification, echo guiding during transcatheter PVL closure, and online fusion imaging facilitating proper conduct of the procedure.

Other chapters provide critical assessment of the currently available equipment, especially the occluders. Special emphasis is placed on the current techniques used for transvascular and transapical PVL closure. The management of paravalvular leaks after transcatheter aortic valve implantation (TAVI) is also addressed, mainly because of similarities of techniques used for PVL closure. We acknowledge however that TAVI-related PVL might reflect the shortcomings of the first-generation TAVI devices and are of different etiology than those related to surgical valves.

Description of the most common pitfalls in transcatheter PVL treatment is emphasized.

The summary includes remarks on the limitation of the available data and future perspectives.

We hope that the publication of this book will contribute to an increase in the understanding of the problem and will foster international collaboration on the development in this area.

Katowice, Poland   Grzegorz Smolka
                                                                          Wojciech Wojakowski
                                                                             Michal Tendera

Contents

List of Videos

- **Movie 1a and 1b:** Examples of paravalvular leaks (PVLs) with absent (**1a**) or present (**1b**) surgical sutures crossing the lumen (as confirmed with catheter movements after PVL crossing). Note the differences in prosthetic ring mobility despite the similar size of both lesions.
- **Movie 2:** CD-mapped flow across PVL with the identification of true vena contracta (VC) (arrow).
- **Movie 3:** The direction of guidewire extension can be visualized by zoomed RT 3D TEE VR.
- **Movie 4:** The onset of spontaneous echo contrast (SEC) promptly following mitral transcatheter paravalvular leak closure (TPVLC) (**4a** – before TPVLC, **4b** after TPVLC).
- **Movie 5:** Stentless aortic prosthesis - instant clotting of "dead space" as a result of TPVLC (**5a** – before TPVLC, **5b** after TPVLC).

Electronic supplementary material is available in the online version of the related chapter on SpringerLink: http://link.springer.com/

Chapter 1
Surgical Aspects of Paravalvular Leak

Alberto Pozzoli, Ottavio Alfieri, Francesco Maisano, and Maurizio Taramasso

1.1 Preamble

Paravalvular leak (PVL) is a common complication after surgical valve replacement, with reported incidences at follow-up varying from 2% to 17% in both mitral and aortic positions [1–3].

Among patients in whom PVL develops after surgery, approximately 3% require reoperations because of heart failure, hemolysis, or a combination of both [4–6]. Surgical reoperation is the standard treatment for symptomatic PVLs [5, 6]. It has been demonstrated that in symptomatic patients with PVL, surgical treatment is associated with improved survival compared with conservative management [3]. However, redo surgery is often associated with high morbidity and mortality: several series report an acute mortality between 6% and 22% after surgical reoperation for PVL [7]. Increased risk was observed in severely symptomatic patients (NYHA classes III–IV and severe hemolysis) and in patients with multiple surgical reinterventions. Associated co-pathologies could further increase operative risk.

A. Pozzoli • O. Alfieri
San Raffaele University Hospital, Milan, Italy

F. Maisano
UniversitätsSpital Zürich, University of Zürich, Zürich, Switzerland

M. Taramasso, M.D. (✉)
UniversitätsSpital Zürich, University of Zürich, Zürich, Switzerland

University Heart Clinic Zürich, Rämistrasse 100, 8091 Zürich, Switzerland
e-mail: maurizio.taramasso@usz.ch

© Springer Nature Singapore Pte Ltd. 2017
G. Smolka et al. (eds.), *Transcatheter Paravalvular Leak Closure*,
DOI 10.1007/978-981-10-5400-6_1

1.2   Anatomy of the Structures Adjacent to Aortic and Mitral Valves

The interrelationships among the heart valves in normal hearts are remarkably uniform. The aortic valve occupies a central position, wedged between the mitral valve and the tricuspid valve. The pulmonary valve is instead situated anterior, superior, and slightly to the left of the aortic valve. Importantly, the annuli of the mitral and tricuspid valves merge with each other and with the membranous septum to form the fibrous skeleton of the heart. The core is the central fibrous body, with two extensions, the right and the left fibrous trigones. The right fibrous trigone forms a dense junction between the mitral and tricuspid annuli, the left ventricular-aortic junction (below the non-coronary cusp), and the membranous septum. The left fibrous trigone (more anterior and to the left) lies between the left ventricular-aortic junction and the mitral annulus.

For practical reasons, we will treat specifically the surgical anatomy of the aortic and mitral valve annuli. The annulus fibrosus of the mitral valve is not visible from an atrial point of view, and the part where leaflets attach is deeper and located 2 mm posteriorly. Posteriorly is a discontinuous band of connective tissue that exists only in some parts of the attachment of the posterior leaflet. Instead, the annulus does not exist at the attachment of the anterior leaflet because the leaflet tissue is continuous with the aorto-mitral curtain that extends from the aortic valve annulus to the base of the anterior leaflet. The shape of the annulus varies during the cardiac cycle, it is circular during the diastole, and it becomes kidney shaped during the systole, due to the displacement of the aorto-mitral curtain toward the center of the orifice. Of course, pathological processes will alter this normal anatomy.

Four anatomical structures close to the annulus are at risk during surgery: (a) the circumflex artery, which runs posteriorly and could be injured; (b) the coronary sinus, which skirts the attachment of the posterior leaflet; (c) the bundle of His which is located near the right trigone; and (d) the non-coronary and left coronary aortic cusps which are in close relationship with the base of the anterior leaflet (there is a 6–10 mm safety zone for the placement of sutures in this area) (Fig. 1.1). Instead, the annulus of the aortic valve is a well-delineated scallop-shaped fibrous structure firmly attached to the trigones, the aorto-mitral curtain, and the muscular and membranous septa. The aortic annular plane (the plane joining the nadirs of the aortic annulus) forms a 120° angle with the plane of the mitral valve orifice. The scalloped shape of the annulus delineates three commissural tips that attach the leaflet commissures. There are also three subaortic segments, composed of three triangular subcommissural structures, which form the junction between the aortic root and the ventricular outflow tract. The triangle between the right and the non-coronary sinuses includes the membranous septum. The triangle between the non-coronary and the left coronary sinuses is part of the aorto-mitral curtain. The triangle between the right and the left coronary sinuses is muscular at its base and fibrous at its summit (in continuity with the ventricular septum). Four anatomical structures are at risk during aortic valve surgery: (a) the bundle of His, normally located at the junction between the ventricular and membranous septum, in the subcommissural area between the

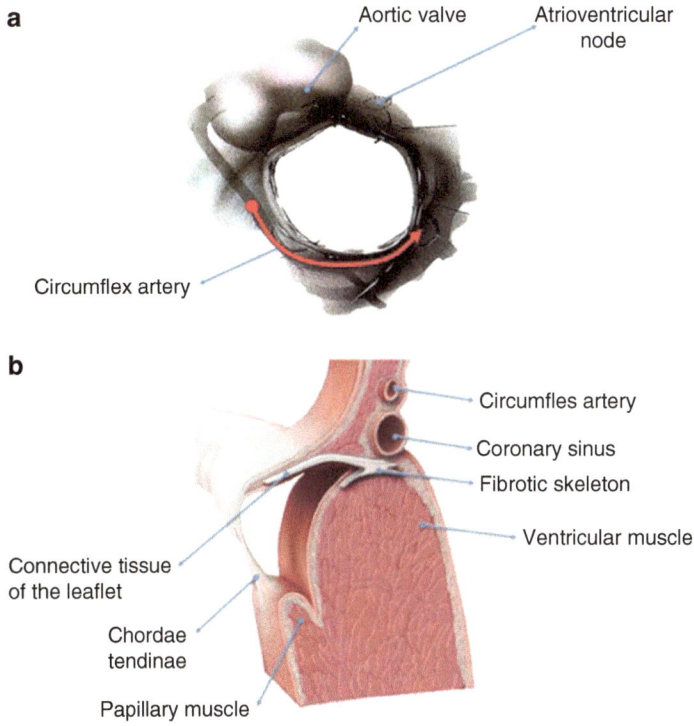

Fig. 1.1 Panel (**a**): anatomical pitfalls during mitral valve surgery. Panel (**b**): section of the mitral valve complex, focusing on the structures which constitute the leaflet, the annulus, and the ventricular muscle

Fig. 1.2 Aortic sinuses, coronary arteries, and the location of the His bundle in respect to the sinuses

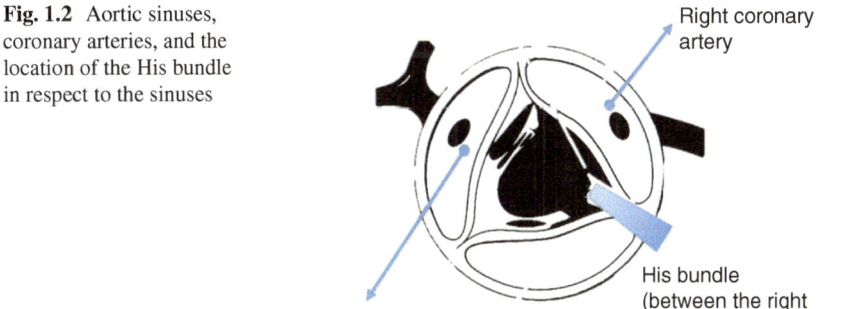

right and the non-coronary sinuses; (b) the membranous septum, due to its fragility, can tear in case of inappropriate surgical bites; (c) the thin proximal part of the aortic sinuses, which can be injured if the surgical stitch is passed very large around the annulus than through it; and (d) the left main coronary artery, due to its proximity to the subcommissural area between the right and the left sinuses (Fig. 1.2).

1.3   Importance of Degeneration or Inflammatory Processes on Stability of Tissues

Unless it is injured, the normal endothelium is resistant to infection by most bacteria and to thrombus formation. Except for those patients in whom the PVLs are caused by technical errors, the other cases are due to an endothelial injury (e.g., at the site of impact of high-velocity jets or on the low-pressure side of a cardiac structural lesion) which causes abnormal flow and allows either direct infection by microorganisms or the development of an uninfected platelet-fibrin thrombus. This thrombus subsequently serves as a site of bacterial attachment during transient bacteremia and will impair tissue stability. The cardiac lesions most commonly associated to this pathological process are mitral regurgitation, aortic stenosis and regurgitation, ventricular septal defects, and complex congenital heart disease. Also, these non-bacterial thrombi can arise as a result of a hypercoagulable state (marantic endocarditis—uninfected vegetations seen in patients with malignancy and chronic diseases) and to bland vegetations complicating autoimmune syndromes, in particular systemic lupus erythematosus and the antiphospholipid antibody syndrome. From a pathological standpoint, those organisms that will cause prostheses detachments due to infections generally reach the bloodstream from mucosal surfaces, the skin, or sites of focal infection. Except for more virulent bacteria (e.g., *S. aureus*) that can adhere directly to intact endothelium or exposed subendothelial tissue, microorganisms in the blood adhere to thrombi and induce a procoagulant state at the site. Although the relationship is not absolute, the causative microorganism is primarily responsible for the temporal course of endocarditis and, thereafter, for injuries between the sewing ring of the prosthesis, the sutures, and the native annulus. Hemolytic streptococci, *S. aureus*, and pneumococci typically result in an acute course, although *S. aureus* occasionally causes subacute disease. Endocarditis caused by Staphylococcus lugdunensis (a coagulase-negative species) or by enterococci may present acutely. Subacute endocarditis is typically caused by viridans streptococci, enterococci, coagulase-negative staphylococci, and the HACEK group (*Haemophilus* species, *Aggregatibacter* species, *Cardiobacterium hominis*, *Eikenella corrodens*, and *Kingella* species) [8].

1.3.1   Surgically Implanted Heart Valves (Types of Prostheses, Different Valve Implantation Positions, Suture Techniques, etc.)

Occurrence of PVL is related to the surgical technique and to endocarditis, usually affecting the sewing ring or the interface of the prosthetic valve and the annulus (often a site of clot formation; Fig. 1.3). It can result in a true detachment of the valve if the lesion is wide. More dramatically, progression of uncontrolled infection

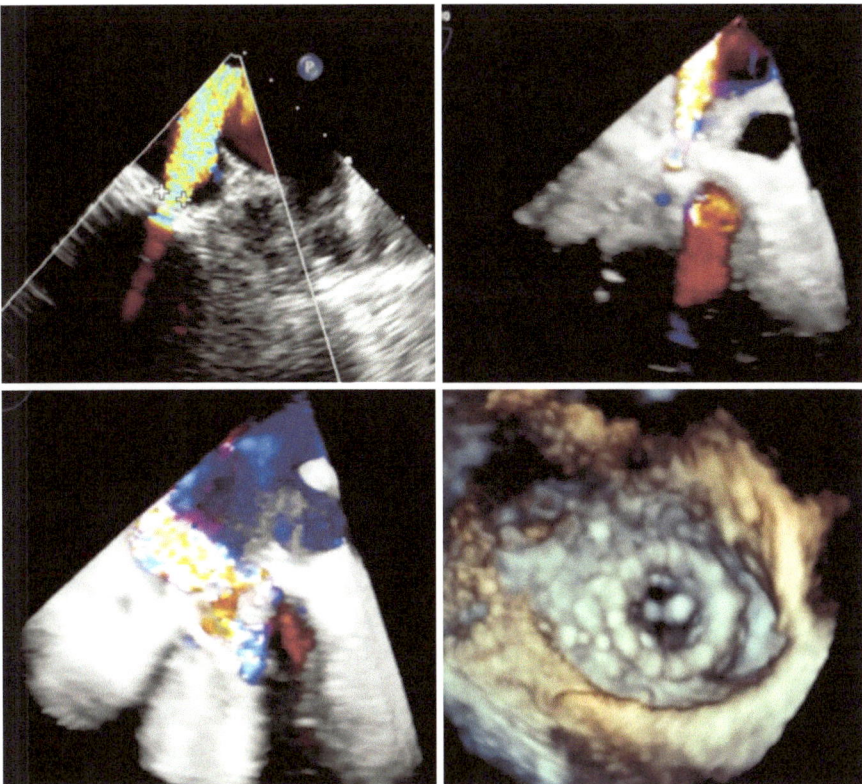

Fig. 1.3 Multiple echocardiographic windows illustrating a perivalvular jet causing severe mitral regurgitation

may lead to perivalvular abscess formation. Occurrence of PVL is related to the surgical technique and to inflammation/endocarditis. With careful annular decalcification and closely placed sutures (pledgeted), these events can be minimized. Above in the text the main techniques used for surgical replacement will be illustrated.

– Aortic Valve Replacement

During the operation the leaflets of the aortic valve are excised to the level of the annulus, and the annulus is thoroughly debrided of any calcium. Extensive decalcification is of paramount importance, and this maneuver will minimize the risk of PVL and dehiscence, particularly in those patients implanting prostheses with thinner sewing rings (Fig. 1.4). More, it will allow for better seating of the valve prosthesis. In most cases, to replace the aortic valve, the annulus is encircled by three 2-0 prolene sutures. Alternatively, multiple single-braided 2-0 sutures may be placed, extending from the aortic to the ventricular surface (everting). Importantly, there could be an anatomic predisposition to periprosthetic leak in

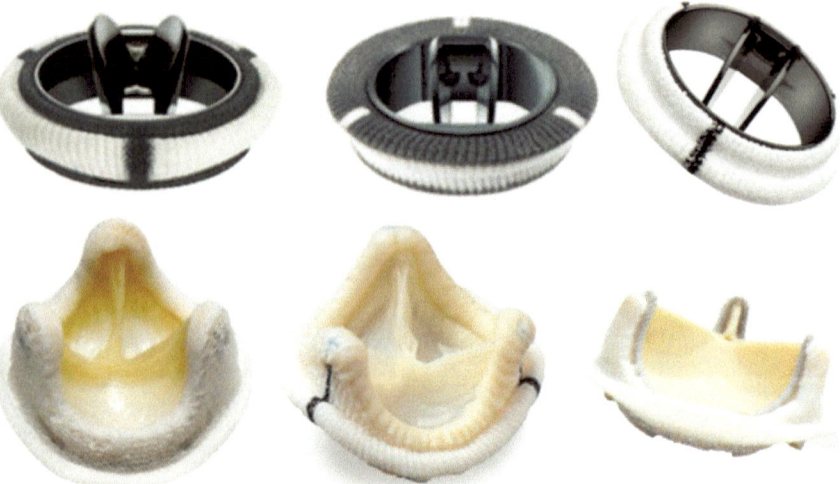

Fig. 1.4 Wide variation between mechanical and tissue prostheses when the sewing cuff is considered

the area of the annulus extending from the right and non-coronary commissure, one-third the distance along the right coronary cusp, and two-thirds the distance to the non-coronary cusp, due to intrinsic weakness in this area of the annulus [9]. The current range of aortic PVL is less than 1% per patient-year, with early postoperative occurrence predominating.

– Mitral Valve Replacement

Analyzing the surgical techniques adoptable during the first operation, suturing techniques vary according to the type of mitral prosthesis implanted. The strongest type of suturing technique to the mitral annulus is the one which places the sutures from the ventricle to the atrium (noneverting or subannular) [10]. To ensure adequate function of bileaflet valves, everting sutures (atrium to ventricle to sewing ring) could also be adopted. This technique pushes the prosthetic valve out into the center of the orifice and minimizes any tissue interference of the prosthetic valve leaflets. This is important when the subvalvular apparatus is preserved. Teflon pledgeted sutures, particularly with the thin sewing rings of the currently bileaflet mechanical valves, are advised. Alternatively, a running prolene suture for implantation of mitral valves is the other technique of choice. Although this technique makes a very clean suture line with minimal knots, it has an increased risk of valve dehiscence if an infection occurs [11]. Because of improved surgical techniques and the use of Teflon pledgets, the incidence of PVLs has fallen from below 1.5% per patient-year, without any differences for both mechanical and biologic prostheses [3, 12]. Historically, PVL was slightly more common with the bileaflet valve than with the porcine valve because of the need for the everting suture technique and less bulky sewing ring [13, 14].

1.3.1.1 Factors Influencing Valve Detachment (Creation of Paravalvular Leaks)

The incidence of PVL for both mechanical and biologic valves is about 0–1.5% per patient-year. The PVLs are the result of an incomplete seal between the sewing ring and annulus. This may arise from abnormal pressure or traction forces on the prosthesis occurring after surgery [9, 15]. Several factors are known to increase the risk of PVL formation [16, 17]. They include annular calcification, infection, suturing technique, as well as the size and shape of prosthetic implant. The early occurrence of PVLs is usually associated with the technical aspects of the surgical implant. Late PVLs are commonly a consequence of suture dehiscence caused by endocarditis or the gradual disruption of incompletely debrided annular calcifications. The regurgitant flow across the perivalvular area frequently leads to hemolysis and, as discussed previously, through denuding of the endocardium to PVE. The number of cases of PVE is on the rise as the number of patients with prosthetic heart valves continues to increase, with an incidence of early PVE around 1% and an incidence of late PVE (after 1 month from operation) slightly inferior, 0.5–1% per year [18]. The risk of PVE appears to be greatest at approximately 5 weeks following valve implantation and thereafter declines [19]. According to the literature, the type of prosthesis (mechanical versus bioprosthetic) does not influence the risk of PVE. Early PVE is usually the result of intraoperative infection (common portals of entry for bacteria causing PVE are intravascular catheters and skin infection). Nosocomial infections contribute to late PVE, particularly in patients with medical comorbidities that require frequent hospital admission or instrumentation (e.g., hemodialysis patients) or immunosuppression (e.g., organ transplantation) [8].

Because of the highly invasive nature of PVE, around 40% of affected patients merit surgical treatment. In the case of perivalvular infections, a complication which occurs in 45–60% of prosthetic valve infections is suggested by persistent unexplained fever during appropriate therapy. Extension can occur from any valve but is most common with aortic valve infection. TEE with color Doppler is the test of choice to detect perivalvular abscesses (sensitivity more than 85%). Although occasional perivalvular infections are cured medically, surgery is warranted when fever persists, fistulae develop, prostheses are dehisced and unstable, and invasive infection relapses after appropriate treatment.

1.3.1.2 Surgical Treatment of Paravalvular Leaks (Techniques, Efficacy of Surgical Treatment, Clinical Trials, Registries)

Although for redo surgery median sternotomy remains the approach of choice, the right anterolateral thoracotomy approach could be an alternative in selected patients (e.g., patent bypass grafts on the left system). It is a safe alternative for mitral valve replacement, because it provides excellent exposure of the mitral valve with minimal need for dissection within the pericardium.

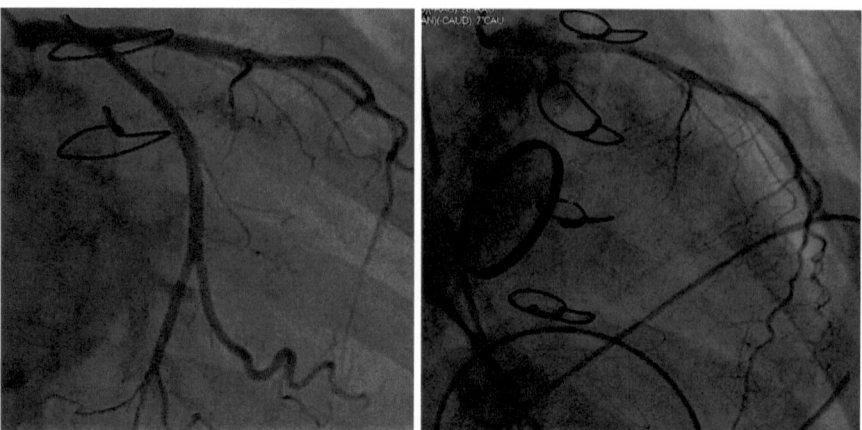

Fig. 1.5 Accidental occlusion of the circumflex artery after surgical mitral valve replacement. *Red dots* trace the occluded vessel on the *right* panel

When evaluating patients with a PVL, an assessment of valve function is mandatory. If the valve itself is competent, direct repair of the leak avoids the hazards of valve replacement. While pledgeted suturing may be attempted for smaller leaks, fibrotic tethering of surrounding tissue and the size of the defect may require a bovine or autologous pericardial patch. In cases of significant dehiscence or associated valvular dysfunction, removal of the valve is necessary. However, in this situation, valve replacement is prone to leak recurrence because the annulus is partially intact, often calcified, and otherwise less than ideal for suture placement. In this context, accidental injury of the circumflex artery could happen (Fig. 1.5). A bovine pericardial skirt can be fashioned and sewn to the sewing ring of the valve. Annular sutures then are placed in a typical fashion through the sewing ring, and the valve is seated.

– Reconstruction of the Mitral Annulus

Once exposure of the mitral valve is obtained, the infected prosthesis is removed. Mitral valve PVE may produce an abscess cavity separating the left atrium, left ventricle, and prosthesis. In these situations the operation includes debridement of the annulus with subsequent annulus reconstruction using autologous or glutaraldehyde-fixed bovine pericardium (David technique) [20]. With this technique, a semicircular pericardial patch is used to reconstruct the annulus with one side of the patch sutured to the endocardium of the left ventricle and the other side to the left atrium. This patch closes off the cavity, which must be thoroughly debrided before the patch is affixed. The new valve prosthesis is affixed to this reconstructed annulus. In most situations with annular reconstruction, a bioprosthesis is favorably employed because of the larger and softer sewing ring and to avoid anticoagulation in the postoperative period.

– Reconstruction of the Fibrous Trigones

Extension of infection into the intervalvular fibrosa/fibrous trigones may necessitate replacement of both mitral and aortic valves. This usually occurs in the setting of PVE affecting both the aortic and the mitral valves and seldom with isolated mitral valve endocarditis [21]. Reconstruction of the intervalvular fibrosa and replacement of both the aortic and mitral valve are required. In such circumstances the fibrous trigones may be reconstructed with autologous or bovine pericardium that is used to secure the new prosthesis [19]. Perfect exposure is mandatory whether it is provided by the extended transseptal approach or by dividing the superior vena cava and extending the left atriotomy from the anterior to the right superior pulmonary vein toward the dome of the left atrium. This approach allows debridement of both the aortic and mitral valves, as well as the fibrous trigones. The prosthetic mitral valve is then sewn to the annulus posteriorly, medially, and laterally, and the superior portion of the mitral valve annulus is reconstructed with a pericardial patch that replaces the fibrous trigones. The valve is then sewn to the patch with horizontal mattress sutures. Once the mitral valve is secured in place, the aortic valve prosthesis is affixed to the aortic annulus. The pericardial patch is used to reconstruct the medial part of the aortic valve annulus. The aortic valve is then sewn to that patch [19]. An alternative option is aortic valve and root replacement in an anatomic position, suturing the intervalvular fibrosa/mitral valve of the homograft to the mitral valve prosthesis.

Limited data exist on the long-term surgical outcomes to treat PVLs. Redo surgery in this context is often associated with high morbidity and mortality rates, as well as a high risk of leak recurrence [1]. Surgical reoperation is the standard treatment for symptomatic PVLs [3–6]. It has been demonstrated that in symptomatic patients with PVL, surgical correction is associated with an improved survival compared with conservative management. Increased risk was observed in severely symptomatic patients (NYHA classes III–IV and severe hemolysis) and in patients with multiple surgical reinterventions. Associated co-pathologies could further increase operative risk. Several series report an acute mortality between 6% and 22% after surgical reoperation for PVL [3–7]. To date, long-term longitudinal outcomes after surgical treatment of PVL are largely unknown. Taramasso et al. reported the long-term results (up to 14 years) of the surgical treatment of PVL of a large series of patients from a single high-volume center experience [22]. Patients with mitral PVL were in slightly worse baseline clinical condition and were significantly more symptomatic compared with patients with aortic PVL. This study confirmed that surgery is an effective option for the treatment of PVL. Intraprocedural success was 98%, and in patients with wide and multiple leaks, it was possible to achieve optimal anatomic results. Of note, redo surgery for recurrent PVL was required during follow-up in a single case. However, in the absence of a rigorous echocardiographic follow-up, freedom from reoperation may underestimate the rate of PVL recurrence, because many patients with recurrence could not have undergone reoperation because of the prohibitive risk of redo surgery. In regard to safety, the 30-day mortality reported in this study is relatively high (>10%, all cardiac-related deaths), confirming that surgery in the context of patients with PVL is still a high-risk procedure. Patients with PVL are usually patients with multiple previous open operations, with associated co-pathologies and severely symptomatic. In view of the high-risk profile of the patients included in the series, a 10% of acute mortality may be considered acceptable, being comparable to that reported in other surgical series. It was not identified in any specific subgroup of patients with significantly higher risk for acute mortality. A trend toward a higher mortality in mitral patients was observed, reflecting the more compromised clinical conditions of the patients with mitral PVL. The most important finding of literature revision is that long-term results of conventional surgery in the context of PVLs are largely suboptimal [1–3, 9, 16, 22]. In the experience of San Raffaele University Hospital, overall actuarial survival at 12 years was less than 40%, and this is particularly significant considering the relatively young age of the patients included in the study (<62 years on average) [22]. This aspect may be partially explained by the high-risk preoperative profile. In particular, preoperative chronic renal failure and the presence of more than one previous cardiac operation were independently associated with increased risk of mortality at follow-up. Patients with mitral PVL had a higher cardiac-related mortality at follow-up compared with patients with aortic PVL. Although preoperative left ventricular ejection fraction was preserved in both aortic and mitral PVL cases, patients with mitral valve disease more frequently have a certain degree of associated left ventricular dysfunction that could affect long-term outcomes. Moreover, the natural history of patients with a prosthetic valve in the mitral position is usually worse if compared with the natural course of patients with an aortic prosthesis [1]. The high 30-day mortality and the disappointing long-term results that we observed strongly point out the need for a valid therapeutic option alternative to conventional surgery, mainly in the patients presenting with risk factors for increased mortality (patients with multiple previous cardiac operation, associated chronic renal failure, and mitral PVL). Percutaneous PVL closure has been proposed as an attractive less invasive option and was found to alleviate the consequences and symptoms of PVLs in high-risk patients [23]. Transcatheter closure of PVLs with different approaches is an emerging and challenging field, with promising initial results [24]. However, percutaneous PVL closure requires very experienced and skilled operators. Reproducibility currently remains a major concern: technical success rates range from 60% to 90% in different series [25]. The integration of conventional surgery and transcatheter closure may reduce the global mortality, offering the unique opportunity of a real patient-tailored approach.

References

1. Hammermeister K, Sethi GK, Henderson WG, Grover FL, Oprian C, Rahimtoola SH. Outcomes 15 years after valve replacement with a mechanical versus a bioprosthetic valve: final report of the Veterans Affairs randomized trial. J Am Coll Cardiol. 2000;36:1152–8.
2. Ionescu A, Fraser AG, Butchart EG. Prevalence and clinical significance of incidental paraprosthetic valvar regurgitation: a prospective study using transoesophageal echocardiography. Heart. 2003;89:1316–21.
3. Genoni M, Franzen D, Vogt P, Seifert B, Jenni R, Künzli A, et al. Paravalvular leakage after mitral valve replacement: improved long-term survival with aggressive surgery? Eur J Cardiothorac Surg. 2000;17:14–9.
4. Nishida T, Sonoda H, Oishi Y, Tanoue Y, Nakashima A, Shiokawa Y, et al. Single- institution, 22-year follow-up of 786 CarboMedics mechanical valves used for both primary surgery and reoperation. J Thorac Cardiovasc Surg. 2014;147:1493–8.

5. Jindani A, Neville EM, Venn G, Williams BT. Paraprosthetic leak: a complication of cardiac valve replacement. J Cardiovasc Surg. 1991;32:503–8.
6. Miller DL, Morris JJ, Schaff HV, Mullany CJ, Nishimura RA, Orszulak TA. Reoperation for aortic valve periprosthetic leakage: identification of patients at risk and results of operation. J Heart Valve Dis. 1995;4:160–5.
7. LaPar DJ, Yang Z, Stukenborg GJ, Peeler BB, Kern JA, Kron IL, et al. Outcomes of reoperative aortic valve replacement after previous sternotomy. J Thorac Cardiovasc Surg. 2010;139:263–72.
8. Kasper DL, Fauci AS, Longo DL, Hauser SL, Larry Jameson J, Loscalzo J, editors. Harrison's principles of internal medicine. 19th ed. New York: McGraw-Hill Medical; 2015.
9. De Cicco G, Lorusso R, Colli A, et al. Aortic valve periprosthetic leakage, anatomic observations and surgical results. Ann Thorac Surg. 2005;79:1480.
10. Chambers EP Jr, Heath BJ. Comparison of supra-annular and subannular pledgeted sutures in mitral valve replacement. Ann Thorac Surg. 1991;51:60. discussion 63
11. Dhasmana JP, Blackstone EH, Kirklin JW, Kouchoukos NT. Factors associated with periprosthetic leakage following primary mitral valve replacement: with special consideration of the suture technique. Ann Thorac Surg. 1983;35:170.
12. Torregrosa S, Gomez-Plana J, Valera FJ, et al. Long-term clinical experience with the Omnicarbon prosthetic valve. Ann Thorac Surg. 1999;68:881.
13. Burckhardt D, Striebel D, Vogt S, et al. Heart valve replacement with St Jude Medical valve prosthesis: long-term experience in 743 patients in Switzerland. Circulation. 1988;78:I18–24.
14. Gallucci V, Mazzucco A, Bortolotti U, et al. The standard Hancock porcine bioprosthesis: overall experience at the University of Padova. J Card Surg. 1988;3:337.
15. De Cicco G, Russo C, Moreo A, Beghi C, Fucci C, Gerometta P, et al. Mitral valve periprosthetic leakage: anatomical observations in 135 patients from a multicenter study. Eur J Cardiothorac Surg. 2006;30:887–91.
16. Rallidis LS, Moyssakis IE, Ikonomidis I, Nihoyannopoulos P. Natural history of early aortic paraprosthetic regurgitation: a five-year follow-up. Am Heart J. 1999;138:351–7.
17. Wasowicz M, Meineri M, Djaiani G, Mitsakakis N, Hegazi N, Xu W, et al. Early complications and immediate postoperative outcomes of paravalvular leaks after valve replacement surgery. J Cardiothorac Vasc Anesth. 2011;25:610–4.
18. Gordon SM, Serkey JM, Longworth DL, et al. Early onset prosthetic valve endocarditis: the Cleveland Clinic experience 1992–1997. Ann Thorac Surg. 2000;69:1388.
19. Lytle BW, Priest BP, Taylor PC, et al. Surgical treatment of prosthetic valve endocarditis. J Thorac Cardiovasc Surg. 1996;111:198.
20. David TE, Feindel CM. Reconstruction of the mitral annulus. A ten-year experience. J Thorac Cardiovasc Surg. 1995;110:1323.
21. David TE. The surgical treatment of patients with prosthetic valve endocarditis. Semin Thorac Cardiovasc Surg 1995;7:47.
22. Taramasso M, Maisano F, Denti P, Guidotti A, Sticchi A, Pozzoli A, et al. Surgical treatment of paravalvular leak: long-term results in a single-center experience (up to 14 years). J Thorac Cardiovasc Surg. 2015;149(5):1270–5.
23. Hourihan M, Perry SB, Mandell VS, Keane JF, Rome JJ, Bittl JA, et al. Transcatheter umbrella closure of valvular and paravalvular leaks. J Am Coll Cardiol. 1992;20:1371–7.
24. Taramasso M, Maisano F, Latib A, Denti P, Guidotti A, Sticchi A, et al. Conventional surgery and transcatheter closure via surgical transapical approach for paravalvular leak repair in high-risk patients: results from a single-centre experience. Eur Heart J Cardiovasc Imaging. 2014;15:1161–7.
25. Binder RK, Webb JG. Percutaneous mitral and aortic paravalvular leak repair: indications, current application, and future directions. Curr Cardiol Rep. 2013;15:342.

Chapter 2
The Role of Imaging in Paravalvular Leak Assessment

David del Val Martín and Jose Luis Zamorano Gómez

2.1 Introduction

Paravalvular leaks (PVLs), defined as abnormal retrograde communication between the cardiac chambers adjacent to a prosthetic valve, are a relatively uncommon complication associated with valve replacement. Although real prevalence is unknown and differs widely among different studies, the presence of a certain degree of paravalvular regurgitation is not infrequent after prosthetic valve implantation, with an overall reported incidence of 47%. However, the prevalence of significant PVL with potential clinical consequences is estimated between 1 and 12%. Some studies have demonstrated a higher incidence of PVL after surgical mitral valve replacement (2–12%) than following surgical aortic valve replacement (1–5%). Furthermore, the exponential growth of technology in the field of percutaneous valve replacement, especially the well-established use of transcatheter aortic valve replacement (TAVR), has been associated with an increased risk of PVL with an incidence up to 17%. In contrast, PVLs are rarely detected in the pulmonary or tricuspid position [1–8].

Infectious endocarditis, size and shape of annulus, suture loosening, tissue friability, annular fibrosis and calcification leading to an incomplete contact between sewing ring and annulus are typically associated with the appearance of PVL [9].

There are numerous cardiac prosthetic valves available. They may be classified basically in two groups: biological and mechanical valves. Mechanical valves include monoleaflet and bileaflet valves. Biological valves include porcine and pericardial bovine valves, which can be stentless or contain a metal ring or metal struts. PVL is most frequent in mechanical valves but can also occur in bioprosthetic

D. del Val Martín • J.L.Z. Gómez (✉)
Cardiology Department, University Hospital Ramón y Cajal, Madrid, Spain
e-mail: zamorano@secardiologia.es

© Springer Nature Singapore Pte Ltd. 2017
G. Smolka et al. (eds.), *Transcatheter Paravalvular Leak Closure*,
DOI 10.1007/978-981-10-5400-6_2

valves. Immediately after prosthetic valve implantation, a small degree of paravalvular regurgitation may be normal and usually does not have long-term clinical consequences. In general, causes related to the surgical procedure are commonly associated with early PVL, whereas infectious-related causes are more frequent in late PVL [10–13].

Clinical manifestations of PVL vary widely among patients, depending mainly on the severity of the regurgitation. Many patients with mild and haemodynamically non-significant PVL remain asymptomatic, follow a benign clinical course and do not require further intervention. In contrast, patients with severe PVL could present with overt clinical symptoms, which can eventually lead to life-threatening consequences [10, 14].

At present, echocardiography remains the gold standard imaging modality to evaluate cardiac heart valves and to assess prosthetic valve function.

2.2   Clinical Manifestations

Initial diagnosis of PVL can be challenging, and clinical presentation of patients with PVL depends mainly on the severity of the regurgitation. Mitral PVLs are more frequently symptomatic.

Auscultation should be the first approach in patients with suspected PVL. The presence of a new cardiac murmur in patients with a prosthetic valve should trigger the suspicion of PVL. In aortic PVL, a high-pitched diastolic murmur at the left sternal border can be heard. In mitral PVL a holosystolic murmur over left sternal border can be appreciated. However, murmurs are frequently soft and may consequently be undetected [9, 15, 16].

Patients with symptomatic PVLs present typically with congestive heart failure (CHF) and haemolytic anaemia. Pathophysiologically, paravalvular regurgitation behaves similarly to other native valve regurgitation. In mitral PVL, during systole part of the stroke, volume is ejected into a low-pressure chamber (left atrium) using an abnormal low-resistance communication between left ventricle and left atrium. Therefore, haemodynamically significant PVL causes an increased volume overload in the left atrium that may lead to its dilation and congestive heart failure with high pulmonary pressure and pulmonary oedema. In contrast, with mitral PVL, in aortic paravalvular regurgitation, the entire left ventricle stroke volume is ejected into a high-pressure chamber, and diastolic regurgitant flow causes a left ventricular volume overload that can lead to adverse left ventricular remodelling due to high end-systolic and end-diastolic volumes, eventually leading to a decrease in ejection fraction. Congestive heart failure is the most frequent clinical manifestation in symptomatic patients. The severity of symptoms is correlated with the orifice size and the regurgitation volume of PVL, especially in mitral position. The majority of patients with severe PVL present with a New York Heart Association (NYHA) functional class ≥III. Physical examination may reveal signs of congestive heart failure with lower-extremity oedema, jugular venous distention and crackles across lung fields.

The presence of haemolytic anaemia, due to red blood cell destruction secondary to an increased turbulence around regurgitant orifice, is observed in around 30–75% of symptomatic patients and is frequently associated with congestive heart failure symptoms. Haemolysis can be identified by a serum lactate dehydrogenase level > 460 U/L and any two of the three following criteria: blood haemoglobin <13.8 g/dL for males or <12.4 g/dL for females, serum haptoglobin <50 mg/dL and reticulocyte count >2%. The detection of schistocytes in the peripheral blood is an important finding that supports the diagnosis of haemolytic anaemia [17].

The presence of symptoms, either CHF or haemolytic anaemia, is associated with an increased mortality in patients with PVL [16]. Although optimal medical treatment for CHF and periodic blood transfusion in addition to erythropoietin-stimulating agents may be enough to relieve symptoms, some patients remain symptomatic during follow-up. In these patients, surgery may be an adequate solution; however, it is essential to keep in mind that reoperation is associated with a non-negligible inherent morbidity and mortality risk. Since 1992, when percutaneous closure of PVL was first reported by Hourihan et al. [18], a non-invasive approach has emerged as an alternative to open heart surgery, with an encouraging rate of procedural success and good clinical outcomes.

2.3   Imaging Approach of Paravalvular Leaks

2.3.1   Basic Principles

Imaging modalities, especially echocardiography, are the gold standard for the assessment of native cardiac valves due to its wide availability, low cost, versatility, radiation-free and diagnosis accuracy. In the same way, echocardiography is the mainstay tool for the evaluation of prosthetic heart valves. Leaks are defined by echocardiography as echo dropout areas outside the sewing ring confirmed by colour Doppler. However, the echocardiography approach for the assessment of prosthetic heart valves has significant limitations, especially with mechanical valves but also with bioprosthetic valves:

– There are many different types of prosthetic valves with different designs that determinate variations in flow characteristics and in haemodynamic parameters.
– Reverberation, colour artefacts and acoustic shadowing with non-evaluable zones make the assessment of prosthetic valve more challenging.

Initially, in patients with the clinical suspicion of PVLs, the first approach is commonly performed with transthoracic echocardiography (TTE). However, the limitations mentioned above regarding the assessment of prosthetic valve heart make the detection of prosthetic regurgitation difficult, and even the most carefully performed TTE has a sensitivity limit, especially for the mitral position. Furthermore, localization of PVLs using TTE can be technically difficult, and severity assessments of PVLs using TTE are generally much more complex than native valve regurgitation. The eccentric nature of most PVL regurgitation jets with unusual directions makes the application of routine parameters for the assessment of regurgitation severity in native valves difficult. Therefore, many PVLs may be significantly underestimated using TTE, and transesophageal echocardiography (TOE) may be required for accurate definition and quantification of the regurgitation severity.

It should be noted that negative TTE findings do not rule out the presence of PVL (low negative predictive value) and that, in the presence of suggestive clinical presentation or incongruent symptoms and TTE findings, another imaging technique should be performed.

2.3.2 Transthoracic Echocardiography

The approach to identifying a prosthesis regurgitation is similar to native valves and requires the assessment of multiple colour Doppler flow imaging and Doppler echocardiographic parameters.

First of all, a two-dimensional echocardiography imaging (2D-TTE) comprehensive assessment should be performed for the evaluation of prosthetic valve characteristics (bileaflet, monoleaflet or caged-ball mechanical valves or bioprosthetic valves) with special emphasis in prosthetic valve leaflet morphology, mobility and its position in the sewing ring. Additional information regarding other echocardiographic indirect signs, such as left ventricle size, hypertrophy, systolic function, pulmonary artery pressures, other valve morphology and function, should be assessed. It is essential to compare these measurements with previous TTE examinations because, frequently, slight variations in measures are the first sign of suspicion of haemodynamically significant prosthesis valve regurgitation.

TTE colour Doppler flow imaging can be helpful for the detection of prosthetic valve regurgitation. It is important to note that mechanical prosthesis indeed may have a small degree of physiological regurgitation jets known as leakage backflow, with a washing effect that reduce blood stasis around prosthesis and virtually minimize the risk of thrombus formation. These leakage flows are characterized by being narrow, short in duration, transvalvular and symmetric, and patterns and number of regurgitation jets vary depending on the fluid dynamics of each valve type. Therefore, it is essential to distinguish PVLs from physiological transvalvular regurgitation flows.

For the detection of prosthetic aortic valve regurgitation, TTE is often enough because, generally, it provides a good visualization of left ventricle outflow tract region without intercepting the valve prosthesis and avoiding the limitation of acoustic shadowing. Parasternal long-axis and short-axis views, the apical views and the five-chamber view are appropriate for the detection of PVLs in aortic position. Occasionally, off-axis views may be helpful in determining the origin of the jets. In some cases, aortic regurgitation jets can be undetected using TTE, especially for posterior located PVLs in the non-coronary sinus region, in which regurgitation jets are often shadowed by the prosthesis valve. In these cases, in the presence of clinical suspicion, TOE should be performed (Fig. 2.1) [19, 20].

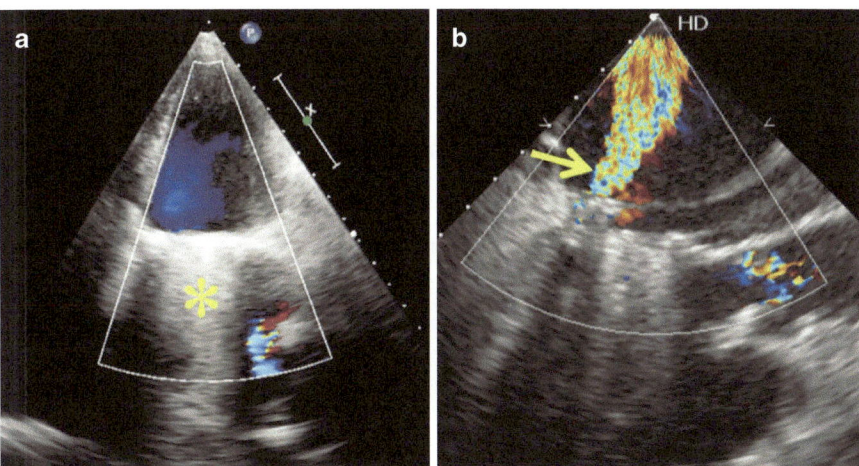

Fig. 2.1 Mitral PVL assess using TTE (**a**) and TOE (**b**). It should be note that echocardiography artefacts, especially acoustic shadowing in mechanical prosthesis, may obscure the presence of PVL in TTE examination (*yellow star*). Thus, in the presence of clinical suspicion, TOE should be performed for an accurate assessment of PVL (*yellow arrow*)

For the detection of prosthetic mitral valve regurgitation, TTE assessment is less useful because the left atrium is veiled by the acoustic shadowing of the prosthesis (especially in mechanical prosthesis). The parasternal view may be helpful for the detection of prosthetic mitral regurgitation because the left atrium is not shadowed by the prosthesis. In contrast, apical views are limited because the left atrium is largely occluded by prosthetic artefact; however, PVLs can occasionally be detected. Even the most carefully and accurate TTE assessment have a low sensitivity for the detection of prosthetic mitral regurgitation. Hence, TOE should be performed in the presence of suggestive clinical presentation or pathological prosthetic mitral valve flow suspicion after TTE examination [19–21].

CW Doppler ultrasound signal may be useful for identifying prosthetic regurgitation even when regurgitation jet flows are not visible and pass undetected by TTE. Initially, it is recommended to align the CW Doppler ultrasound beam parallel to anterograde flow direction of the valve and then to scan the sewing ring to detect any potential abnormal regurgitation jet. In the mitral and tricuspid position, the regurgitation signal begins immediately after the closure of the prosthesis and continues during systole up to the onset of anterograde flow in diastole. However, in aortic and pulmonary position, the regurgitation signal is detected in diastole. The accurate analysis of the CW Doppler recording, with especial emphasis on the timing of different flow signals, is essential for correct identification of prosthetic valve regurgitation and its localization. Indirect signs in CW Doppler recording are also helpful for the evaluation of the severity (density and shape of signal compared with anterograde flow, regurgitation flow velocity, duration and morphology). Be aware that, despite the fact that the use of CW Doppler enhances the likelihood of detecting invisible PVLs over TTE colour Doppler, the eccentric nature of PVLs may

make the correct alignment with CW Doppler ultrasound beam difficult, and occasionally PVLs can still go undetected (Fig. 2.2).

It should be noted that even negative findings in a comprehensive examination
using the combination of different TTE tools (2D-TTE imaging, TTE colour
Doppler and CW Doppler signal) does not exclude the presence of prosthetic valve
regurgitation and further studies should be performed.

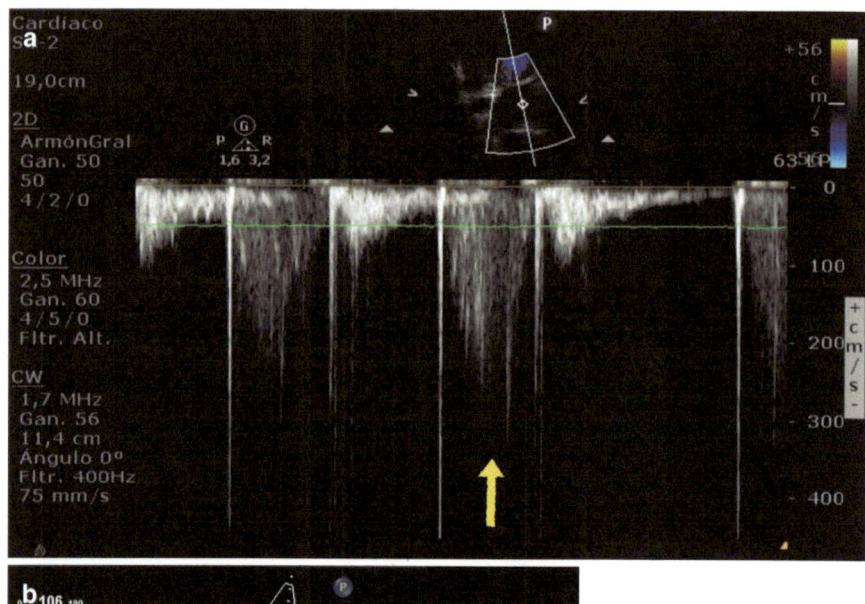

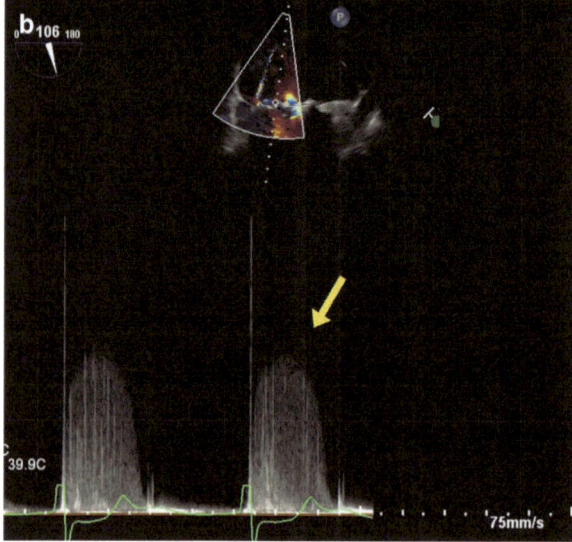

Fig. 2.2 Prosthetic mitral regurgitation. (**a**). TTE four-chamber view and (**b**) TOE four-chamber
view. CW doppler recording of mechanical prosthetic mitral regurgitation. Dense, shape, regurgitation flow velocity, duration and morphology of CW doppler signal can be helpful for the estimation of the severity. In this case, CW doppler signal is not too dense and the outline is not well
defined, suggesting regurgitation is not severe

2.3.3   Transesophageal Echocardiography

TOE is considered the mainstay tool for accurate assessment of PVLs, and it should be systematically performed in the presence of clinical suspicion, even when TTE findings do not identify any pathological prosthetic valve regurgitation.

The main technical limitation of TTE for the assessment of prosthetic valves are echocardiography artefacts, specifically in mechanical prosthesis in mitral position, because the left atrium and, accordingly, regurgitation jets are veiled by acoustic shadowing related to metallic components of the prosthesis. Although TOE provides excellent visualization of left atrial and mitral regurgitation jets, due to the acoustic shadowing which lengthens to the opposite direction, other technical problems such as reverberation and colour Doppler artefacts remain an important limitation with both approaches. Despite this, TOE has been proven to be an important complement to the transthoracic approach in technically difficult studies, and it has become the preferred tool for a more precise assessment of the location and quantification of severity in PVLs. Furthermore, TOE may be useful to identify related aetiological conditions such as the presence of valve endocarditis, prosthetic dehiscences, abscess or masses.

As mentioned above, TTE may often be sufficient and, in some cases, superior to TOE for the detection of aortic prosthetic regurgitation [22, 23]. However, TOE approach may be required in technically difficult TTE examinations or when TTE findings are contradictory. In addition, TOE may be helpful to identify the precise origin and to separate paravalvular from transvalvular leakage flows (Fig. 2.3). It is essential to obtain images in multiple views and multiple planes to ensure complete visualization of the valvular and paravalvular region. Colour Doppler examination should be performed carefully in long-axis view, short-axis view and transgastric views for the detection of PVLs in aortic position. Keep in mind that, in contrast to

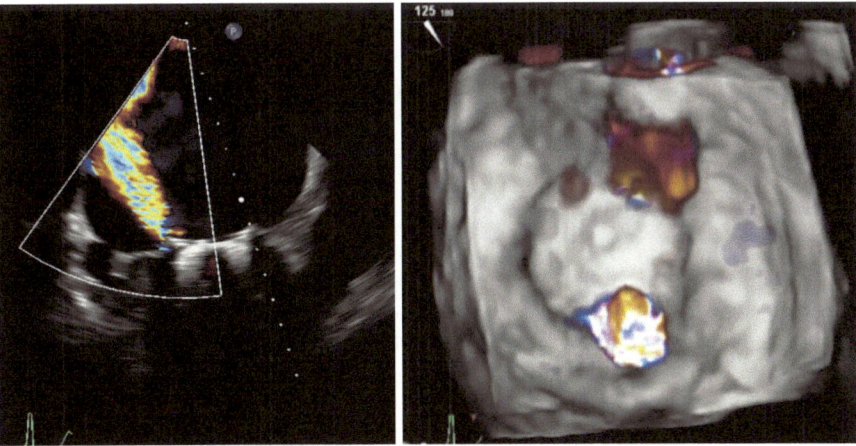

Fig. 2.3 Mitral PVL assess using 2D-TOE and 3D-TOE colour images. It is essential to identify physiologic from pathologic flows and to separate intravalvular and paravalvular jets. In this case, severe paravalvular eccentric jet is visualized with regurgitation origin outside the prosthetic sewing ring

TTE studies, in TOE images, acoustic shadowing of prosthesis affects the anterior region and it may limit the correct evaluation of prosthetic aortic regurgitation at the midesophageal level. Additionally, the presence of concomitant mitral prosthesis may cause significant shadowing and obscure the left ventricular outflow tract, passing unnoticed abnormal flow signals [24–26].

TOE has demonstrated to be superior to TTE in detecting prosthetic mitral regurgitation, and TOE examination is required for its accurate diagnosis [27]. TOE four-chamber view, two-chamber view and long chamber view permit an excellent visualization of the left atrium and the prosthetic sewing ring in order to identify PVLs. A systematic assessment with a detailed scanning of the sewing ring using colour Doppler in multiple angles should be performed to detect prosthetic mitral regurgitation and to distinguish physiologic from pathologic flows and paravalvular from intravalvular regurgitation jets. Typically, in mitral PVLs, when the jet goes through the regurgitant orifice outside the prosthetic ring from the left ventricle to left atrium, the flow tends to be eccentric and adopts unusual directions. Moreover, the role of TOE in mitral PVLs is essential to determine the precise origin and mechanism of the regurgitation jet and to evaluate indirect signs of severity. Among these, systolic flow reversal in pulmonary veins has been correlated with the severity of mitral PVLs, provided that the regurgitation jet is not directed into the interrogated vein.

TOE is also helpful in the good-quality acquisition of other parameters related with regurgitation severity. TOE examination and the use of off-axis views provide a better visualization of PVLs flow throughout its entire length, facilitating the alignment of CW Doppler ultrasound beam and improving the CW Doppler signal. In addition to other parameters, the analysis of CW Doppler recording allows estimation and quantification of the severity of the regurgitation [28].

Importantly, TOE is not only important to identify and define the degree of PVL. Selection of the appropriate treatment strategy in patients with haemodynamically significant PLVs requires an accurate identification of the shape and size of the regurgitant orifice. In light of this, TOE is not only fundamental for the evaluation and procedural planning of PVL, but it is also the key for guidance during the intervention of percutaneous PVL closure or open heart surgery.

2.3.4   3D Echocardiography

Over recent years, technical advancements in imaging have allowed the development of novel tools to enhance diagnostic accuracy and to overcome classic limitations of 2D-TTE and TOE, particularly in heart valvular disease. One of the most relevant contributions has been the emerging of three-dimensional transthoracic (3DTTE) and transesophageal echocardiography (3DTOE) [29, 30].

In the evaluation of prosthetic heart valves, 3D echocardiography, with or without colour Doppler, provides excellent results for diagnosis and characterization of

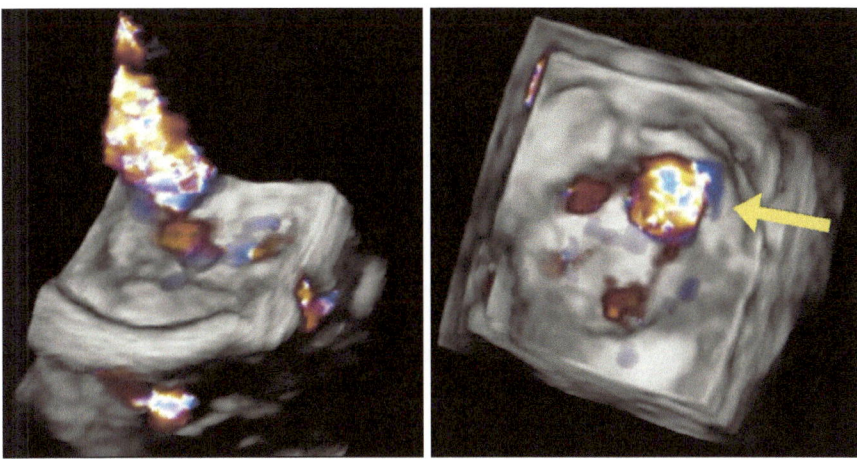

Fig. 2.4 Prosthetic mitral regurgitation. Three-dimensional transesophageal echocardiography color image of mechanical prosthesis. En-face real-time three dimensional colour doppler TOE visualization of the prosthesis also enables to measure the circumferential extent of paravalvular regurgitation that has been associated with the severity of PVL (*yellow arrow*, severe PVL, more than 20% of sewing ring circumference)

all-type prosthetic valve dysfunction, even compared with direct surgical inspection. 3DTTE and more specifically 3D-TOE have been shown to be particularly accurate for the diagnosis of PVLs compared with 2D-TTE. The major advantage of 3DTOE is the capacity to analyse the entire valve in one full volume or 3D zoom instead of the thin slice visualized in 2D echocardiography, providing powerful information about the localization and the extent of regurgitation jets (Fig. 2.4). Also 3DTOE allows the assessment of prosthetic valve details, such as the sewing ring, the leaflet motion and the presence of any PVL etiological conditions (vegetations, abscess, dehiscences) [29–33].

Especially, 3DTOE has been demonstrated an enhancement in the diagnostic accuracy and quantification of regurgitant degree in patients with multiples PVL. The more accurate measurement of flow convergence, vena contracta and the extent of the jet in the receiving chamber permit an improvement of severity quantification. This tool has the ability to acquire a 3D colour full volume that can then be rotated and cropped for the identification and precise delimitation of the effective regurgitant orifice area.

Finally, 3DTEE has been increasingly recognized as invaluable for guidance of procedures for percutaneous PVL closure [34–37].

However, 3DTEE has some limitations indeed. A comprehensive assessment of prosthetic valves can be challenging and technically demanding because it requires high-quality image acquisition. Thus, a complete training process should be carried out by staff of echocardiography laboratories in order to optimize its acquisition.

2.3.5   Intracardiac Echocardiography

In recent years, intracardiac echocardiography (ICE) has become increasingly recognized as a valuable imaging tool for guiding structural heart disease and cardiac arrhythmias procedures. Unlike TOE, it does not require general anaesthesia, which may be especially useful for sick patients in whom local anaesthesia may be more desirable. At present, 2D and 3D intracardiac echocardiography (ICE) represents a complementary technique to other imaging modalities in the assessment of prosthetic valves and more specifically in evaluation of PVL. Its high-image resolution and detail definition provide additional information regarding the severity and the accurate localization and also enable the identification of related causes of PVL: vegetations, abscess or dehiscences [38–40].

Nevertheless, ICE is no stranger to inherent echocardiographic limitations, such as colour artefacts, acoustic shadowing and reverberations that may make an accurate assessment of PVL difficult. Moreover, its invasive nature, the additional costs and the need for specific operator skills remain limitations. For this reason, ICE is not recommended for the first approach in the assessment of PVL.

In current practice, the major role of ICE is the use as intraprocedural guidance of percutaneous PVL closure showing some advantages compared with routine imaging techniques (TOE and fluoroscopy): avoidance of general anaesthesia and reduction of radiation exposure [41].

2.3.6   Stress Echocardiography

Stress echocardiography is a well-established tool for the assessment of patients with valvular heart diseases and suspected prosthetic heart valve dysfunction [42]. Patients with mild or moderate PVL and incongruent exertional symptoms for which the clinical signification is unclear, stress echocardiography may be useful in confirming or excluding the haemodynamically significant repercussion of the paravalvular regurgitation. A symptom-limited grade exercise with supine bicycle and dobutamine stress echocardiography are the most commonly used in most laboratories. Treadmill exercise is occasionally used for the assessment of exercise capacity, but it is less helpful to quantify changes in valvular haemodynamics because the recording of the valve or prosthesis parameters is acquired after completion of exercise, when the haemodynamics may rapidly return to baseline level. In addition to the evaluation of the PVL, other haemodynamically significant findings like inducible ischemia, exercise-induced pulmonary hypertension, impaired left ventricular contractile reserve, dynamic left ventricle dyssynchrony and altered exercise capacity may be assessed [43–46].

A comprehensive assessment of Doppler echocardiographic qualitative or quantitative criteria for prosthetic valve regurgitation severity at rest and during stress echocardiography should be performed. An increase of systolic pulmonary artery pressure up to 60 mmHg during stress echocardiography has been related to the presence of haemodynamically significant mitral regurgitation (intra- or paravalvular) [42, 46, 47]. Occasionally, exercise testing is also helpful to unmask symptoms and to define the optimal timing of intervention in asymptomatic patients with PVL [48, 50].

2.3.7   Cardiac Computed Tomography

Over the last several years, cardiac computed tomography has rapidly emerged as a promising imaging technique for the assessment of prosthetic valves [51]. Recently, preliminary experience concerning the assessment of the role of cardiac CT for detection of complications associated with prosthetic valves, such as thrombosis, pannus formation, suture loosening and endocarditis, has been successfully evaluated with good results.

In recent years, electrocardiography-gated computed tomographic (CT) angiography with three-dimensional (3D) and four-dimensional (4D) reconstruction using volume-rendering techniques has established its usefulness as a reasonable tool for the assessment of PVL. The use of electrocardiography-gated with helicoidal CT acquisition in multiple phases that include the entire cardiac cycle, preferably with retrospective 4D imaging reconstruction, is the protocol recommended for the evaluation of prosthetic PVL; although, the protocol ultimately depends on patients' characteristics, heart rate, CT scanner and CT workstation. In the CT assessment of prosthesis, the main goal is to minimize cardiac and prosthetic movement and to avoid motion artefacts. Hence, it is preferable to use retrospective ECG-gated reconstruction of helical CT acquisition sequences and 4D reconstruction in order to visualize the PVLs in greater detail [52, 55].

Additionally, CT imaging can be helpful in the assessment of the periprosthetic anatomy; structural prosthetic integrity and the surrounding anatomic landmarks, such as the left anterior descending coronary artery course; and the distance between the left ventricular apex and the chest wall (Fig. 2.5) [56, 57, 83].

However, this technique has some drawbacks. Particularly, artefacts from dense structures, such as a prosthetic valve or calcification, may limit PVL size estimation. Furthermore, exposure to radiation and the use of intravenous contrast increase the risks associated with the procedure. Thus, the benefits of high-quality images obtained with this imaging modality should be balanced with the associated risk of radiation, especially in young patients. For this reason, the role of cardiac CT in the evaluation of PVL is mainly to complement echocardiographic findings in order to plan the most suitable treatment rather than purely diagnostic studies.

Therefore, it is important to integrate CT and echocardiographic findings to delimit the detailed localization, size and severity of PVL. At present, both imaging techniques are well-recognized for guidance treatment of PVL [58].

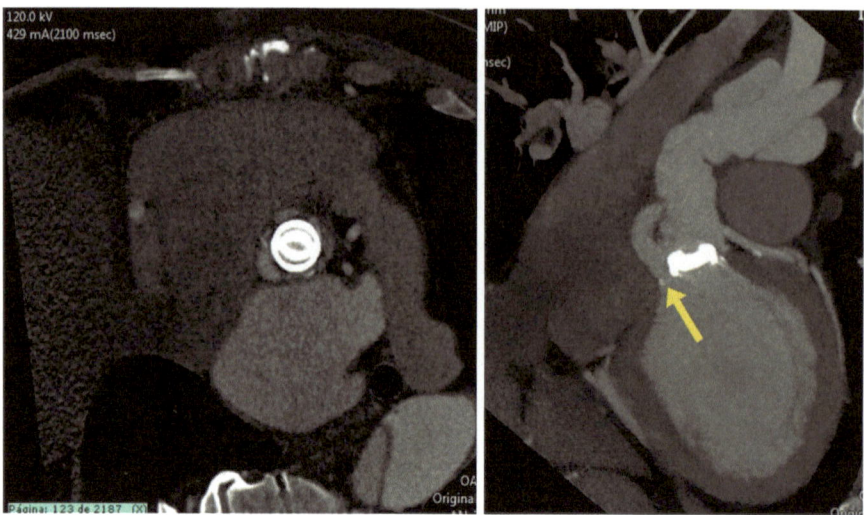

Fig. 2.5 Computed tomography (CT) imaging in prosthetic aortic paravalvular regurgitation. CT imaging provides detailed localization, size and severity of PVL. CT imaging also can be helpful in the assessment of the periprosthetic anatomy, structural prosthetic integrity and the surrounding anatomic landmarks. In these images can be appreciated a PVL (*yellow arrow*) in patient with mechanical aortic prosthesis and ascending aortic dissection

2.3.8   *Cardiac Magnetic Resonance Imaging*

Cardiovascular magnetic resonance (CMR) is an attractive imaging technique for the assessment of cardiac valvular heart disease [59, 60]. CMR provides accurate and reproducible direct quantification of native valvular regurgitation and has been widely recognized as the non-invasive gold standard for quantification of regurgitant volumes. Recently, diverse small studies have demonstrated the feasibility of CMR for evaluation of prosthetic heart valves to complement echocardiography, especially PVL-related transcatheter aortic valve replacement (TAVR) [61–64]. CMR is able to perform accurate flow-imaging and volume-based measurements.

CMR allows direct measurement of regurgitant flow volume that is an important parameter for severity classification. Also, CMR plays an important role in evaluating accurate flow-imaging and volume-based measurements, irrespective of regurgitant jet number or morphology, and in quantifying regurgitant volumes for multiple valve types.

Different CMR sequences are required depending the clinical context and the purpose of the examination. For flow and velocity measurements, phase-contrast sequences can be appropriated, and motion-sensitized acquisitions can be helpful to assess turbulent flow. The development of CMR four-dimensional (4D) flow may provide a comprehensive characterization of flow patterns in the assessment of PVL [65].

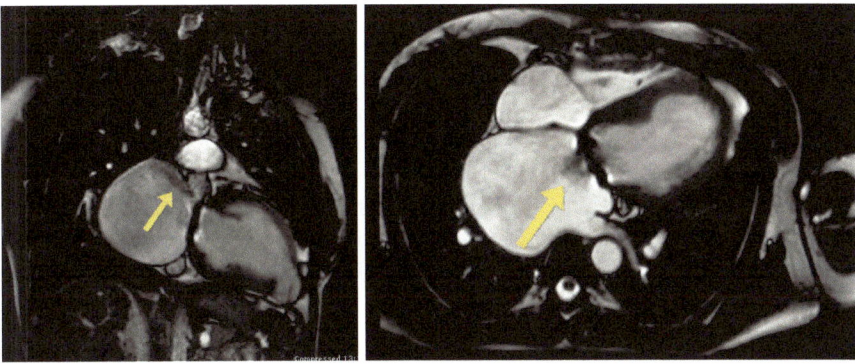

Fig. 2.6 Magnetic resonance imaging in prosthetic mitral regurgitation. Note the presence of systolic flow in left atrium with regurgitant jet origin outside the sewing ring and Coanda effect suggesting significative mitral PVL (*Courtesy Dra. Covadonga Fernández-Golfín, Ramón y Cajal University Hospital. Madrid. Spain*)

CMR assessment of PVL is highly reproducible and complements echocardiographic semiquantitative and quantitative parameters for grading the severity of regurgitation. Importantly, some studies have reported that patients with greater than mild PVL assessed by CMR, with values of regurgitant fraction >20%, present with a higher incidence of adverse events and prognostic implications [66–68].

Although CMR consistently has demonstrated high reproducibility of measurements, this technique also has inherent technical limitations. CMR quantification of volumes requires high-quality images and an experienced operator. Basically, CMR valve-related artefacts depend on the amount of metal. Bileaflet and titanium-containing prosthetic valve cause fewer artefacts than monoleaflet valves or cobalt-chromium alloys. Biological valves containing a simple ring show no disturbing artefacts, unlike valves with metal struts. Additionally, some situations, such as arrhythmias and motion artefacts, may reduce the accuracy of measurement and significantly affect the quality of acquisition. These aspects, in addition to the increased costs and the irregular access to scanners, remain limitations for a widespread use in the assessment of PVL (Fig. 2.6).

2.4   Echocardiography Assessment of Specific Prosthetic PVL

2.4.1   Mitral Paravalvular Regurgitation

Basically, the same methods used for quantifying severity of native mitral valve regurgitation can be applied for prosthetic mitral regurgitation. Nevertheless, it should be noted that many parameters used routinely for quantification of native mitral regurgitation are not specifically validated for the assessment of mitral prosthetic regurgitation, and their application is extrapolated from quantitative parameters in native valve guidelines.

As mentioned, echocardiography is considered the mainstay tool for the diagnosis of mitral PVL. However, a comprehensive assessment of severity of prosthetic mitral regurgitation is frequently challenging. The major limitation in the evaluation of prosthetic mitral valve by echocardiography is the acoustic shadowing that usually obscures regurgitation jets, especially with mechanical prosthesis. This problem is minimized by the use of TOE, which commonly provides an excellent visualization of left atrial and mitral regurgitation jets. Therefore, TOE is the preferred tool for a more precise identification of PVL, and it should be systematically performed when there is TTE or clinical suspicion of pathologic mitral regurgitation.

First of all, it is essential to distinguish intraprosthetic from paraprosthetic regurgitation jets. A thorough evaluation of the entire sewing ring using colour Doppler and a multiple plane echocardiographic approach, sweeping the mitral prosthesis from 0° to 180°, is the key for an accurate identification of mitral PVL.

Following PVL identification it is necessary to define a detailed localization. In order to unify the nomenclature related with localization of PVL around the perimeter of the sewing ring, a clockwise format from a surgeon's perspective is used (mitral valve or mitral prosthesis view from left atrium). In this perspective, the midpoint of the anterior side of the annulus is aligned at the "12 o'clock" position, and the midpoint of the posterior side of the annulus is seen at the "6 o'clock" position. This usually leaves the posterior-medial commissure and interatrial septum approximately at the "3 o'clock" position, while the anterior-lateral commissure and left atrial appendage are seen approximately at the "9 o'clock" position. Anterior location was defined for PVLs situated between 9 and 12 o'clock, septal location for PVLs between 12 and 3 o'clock, posterior location for PVLs between 3 and 6 o'clock and lateral location for PVLs between 6 and 9 o'clock. Some studies and surgical series have revealed that most common localization of mitral PVL is anterior-septal (between 10 and 11 o'clock) and posterior-lateral (between 5 and 6 o'clock) (Fig. 2.7).

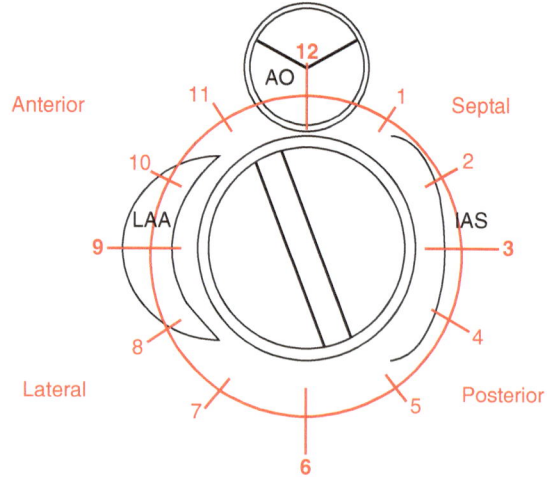

Fig. 2.7 Clockwise format from a surgeon's perspective (mitral valve or mitral prosthesis view from left atrium). In this perspective, the midpoint of the anterior side of the annulus is aligned at the "12 o'clock" position, and the midpoint of the posterior side of the annulus is seen at the "6 o'clock" position (*Courtesy Dr. Eduardo Franco, Ramón y Cajal University Hospital. Madrid. Spain*)

2.4.1.1 Quantification of the Severity of Mitral PVL

Commonly, PVLs in mitral position have a complex morphology, and assessment of the severity of prosthetic mitral paravalvular regurgitation can be difficult. Current recommendations for prosthetic mitral regurgitation assessment, either intra- or paravalvular, are derived from native mitral valvular regurgitation, integrating parameters obtained by different imaging modalities, mainly TTE and TOE. This multi-parametric approach includes findings related to prosthetic valve structure and motion, qualitative or semiquantitative parameters, quantitative parameters and indirect signs. Differentiation of mild from moderate or severe prosthetic PVL is usually easier than discriminating moderate form severe [43–45, 69, 70].

Prosthetic Valve Structure
PVLs are more common with mechanical valves than bioprosthetic valves. An accurate assessment of prosthetic valve structure and motion is required in order to identify abnormal findings related with the severity of mitral PVL. The presence of dehiscence or evidence of valve instability (rocking motion) is associated with significant paravalvular regurgitation. Other findings related with etiological PVL conditions, such as endocarditis, pseudoaneurysm or abscess, are frequently associated with severe mitral PVL and poor clinical prognosis.

Qualitative or Semiquantitative Parameters
Colour Doppler or CW/PW Doppler parameters can point out severity in mitral PVL. Regurgitant jet area can suggest severity of regurgitation. A small thin jet (jet area <4 cm^2) in the left atrium usually reflects mild PVL, while a large, wide jet (>8 cm^2) reflects a moderate or severe regurgitation. Although this parameter can be helpful for the assessment of central regurgitant jets, mitral PVL can be underestimated because regurgitant flow is commonly eccentric and with complex morphology.

The intensity and shape of the PVL CW Doppler signal may also be useful to estimate regurgitant severity. Triangular shape of CW Doppler signal is associated with severe regurgitation. Other qualitative parameters, such as pulmonary venous flow with systolic flow reversal, indicate severe mitral PVL.

The application of the Doppler velocity index (DVI), by using the ratio of the VTIs of the mitral prosthesis to the LV outflow tract (VTI$_{PrMV}$/VTI$_{LVO}$) is an indirect parameter of mechanical mitral prosthetic valve dysfunction. Although it has been widely used as an indirect parameter of prosthetic mitral valve stenosis, the Doppler velocity index may be equally elevated in paravalvular regurgitation (increased mitral inflow and decreased velocity in LVO). DVI values higher than 2.5 are associated with the presence of severe PVL.

Also, the proportion of circumferential extent area of paravalvular regurgitation in relation with the entire prosthetic sewing ring perimeter has been proposed as an appropriate method to estimate the degree of regurgitation, and its application is generally recommended in current guidelines.

Quantitative Parameters
The width of the vena contracta is the quantitative parameter that best relates with angiographic assessment of prosthetic mitral paravalvular regurgitation. Values less than 3 mm reflect mild mitral PVL, whereas values higher than >6 mm are associated

with significant PVL. Moderate mitral PVLs are included in intermediate values of vena contracta width 3–6 mm. Other parameters like regurgitant volume and regurgitant fraction can be useful to separate severe from mild or moderate PVL.

In combination with PVL regurgitation velocity measured by CW Doppler, the radius of the proximal flow convergence can be used to estimate effective regurgitant orifice area (ERO). However, ERO is often over- or underestimated due to the eccentric nature of PVL and the presence of multiple regurgitant jets. Despite the fact that the proximal isovelocity surface area (PISA) has not been specifically validated for PVL quantification, the presence of a large PISA may indicate severe regurgitation.

It should be noted that most of the quantitative parameters used routinely for the assessment of native or prosthetic mitral regurgitation assume effective regurgitant offices (ERO) with spherical shapes. However, the ERO of mitral PVL usually are irregular, and they do not follow any conventional geometrical shape. Therefore, the precise definition of size and shape in mitral PVL are extremely enhanced by using a 3D colour echocardiographic assessment (Fig. 2.8).

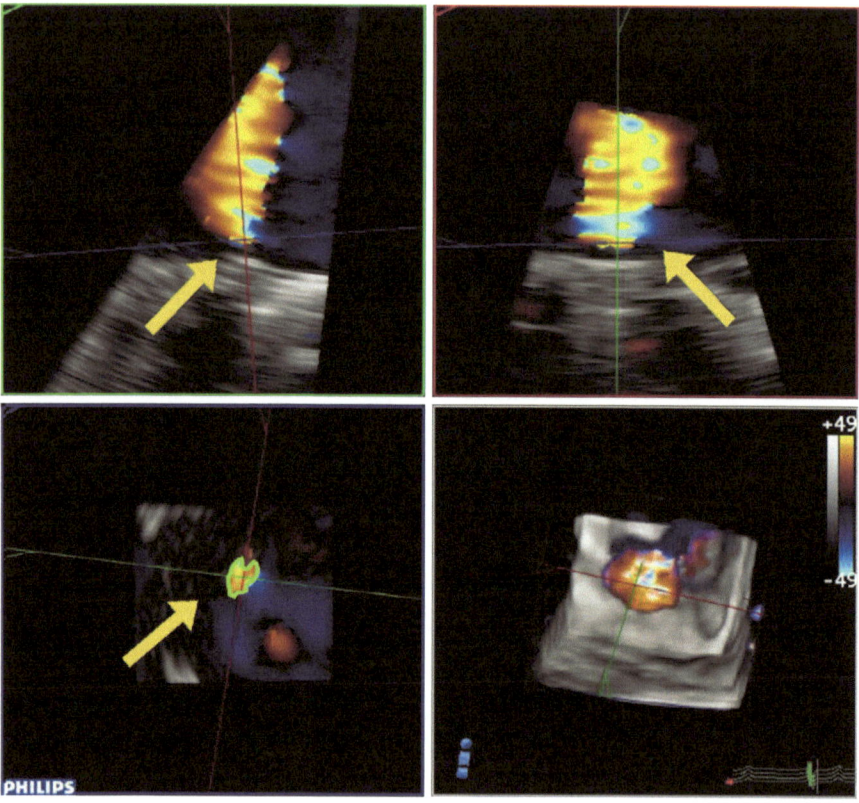

Fig. 2.8 TOE Colour Doppler images and 3D TOE color echocardiographic assessment of mitral paravalvular regurgitation. Commonly, effective regurgitation orifice of mitral PVL is irregular and they do not follow any conventional geometrical shape. 3D colour echocardiographic images provide a high-definition of ERO and allows an accurate measurement of vena contracta (*yellow arrow* and *green line*)

Indirect Sign

Complementarily to direct imaging and Doppler assessment of PVL, additional indirect findings should be evaluated for an overall severity quantification. These indirect signs basically include the size and function of cardiac chambers (left ventricle and left atrial dilatation, left ventricle hypertrophy, systolic function) and the level of systolic pulmonary arterial pressure.

It is grossly important to compare these measurements with previous echocardiographic examination in order to identify slight variations that may reveal novel apparition or worsening of previous PVL (Table 2.1).

Table 2.1 Echocardiographic criteria for severity evaluation of prosthetic mitral valve regurgitation

Mitral	Mild	Moderate	Severe
Valve structural parameters			
Mechanical or bioprosthesis	Usually normal	Usually abnormal	Usually abnormal
Qualitative or semiquantitative parameters			
Colour flow jet area	Small, central jet (usually <4 cm^2 or <20% of LA area)	Variable	Large central jet (usually >8 cm^2 or >40% of LA area) or variable size wall-impinging jet swirling in LA
Flow convergence	None or minimal	Intermediate	Large
Jet density: CW Doppler	Incomplete or faint	Dense	Dense
Jet Contour: CW Doppler	Parabolic	Usually parabolic	Early peaking, triangular
Pulmonary venous flow: PW Doppler	Systolic dominance	Systolic blunting	Systolic flow reversal
Doppler velocity index: PW Doppler	<2.2	2.2–2.5	>2.5
Circumferential extent of paravalvular regurgitation (%)	<10	10–20	>20
Quantitative parameters			
Vena contracta width (mm)	<3	3–6	>6
Regurgitant volume (ml/beat)	<30	30–59	>60
Regurgitant fraction (%)	<30	30–49	>50
Effective regurgitant orifice area (mm^2)	<20	20–39	>40
Indirect signs			
LV size	Normal	Normal/mild dilated	Dilated
LA size	Normal	Normal/mild dilated	Dilated
Pulmonary hypertension (SPAP > 50 mmHg at rest and >60 mmHg at exercise)	Generally absent	Variable	Generally present

Adapted in part from Zoghbi WA, Chambers JB, Dumesnil JG, et al. Recommendations for evaluation of prosthetic valves with echocardiography and Doppler ultrasound. J Am Soc Echocardiogr 2009;22:975–1014

2.4.2 Aortic Paravalvular Regurgitation

Despite the increased use in recent years of complementary imaging modalities, such as CMR and CT, echocardiography remains considered the gold standard technique to assess the severity of aortic PVL.

Several methods can be used to determine the severity of aortic PVL. In general, the same principles guiding the assessment of native aortic valve regurgitation should be followed for quantification of aortic PVL. However, one should be aware that there are very limited data that support the applicability of native aortic valve regurgitation quantitative parameters on aortic PVL, and many of them may be harder to use because of echocardiographic technical limitations mentioned previously.

Trace or mild prosthetic valve regurgitation may be common with both normally functioning mechanical and bioprosthetic aortic prostheses. The first step when prosthetic regurgitation is detected is to identify physiologic from pathologic flows and to separate intravalvular and paravalvular jets. Aortic PVLs jets tend to be eccentric and may flow in unusual directions. In contrast to mitral PVL, TTE is often enough to identify aortic PVL. However, it is highly recommended to perform a TOE examination for an accurate assessment and grading severity.

Secondly, a precise localization and determination of the position along sewing ring circumference is required. A complementary clockwise format from a surgeon's perspective is used for aortic PVL localization. In this view, "3–4 o'clock" position corresponds to the commissure between left and right coronary sinuses, 7–8 o'clock position corresponds to the commissure between the right and non-coronary sinuses and "11 o'clock" position is aligned at the commissure between the left and non-coronary sinuses. This designation usually leaves the midpoint of the left aortic cusp at the "12–1 o'clock" position, the midpoint of the right aortic cusp at the "5 o'clock" position and the midpoint of the non-coronary aortic cups at the "9 o'clock" position (Fig. 2.9).

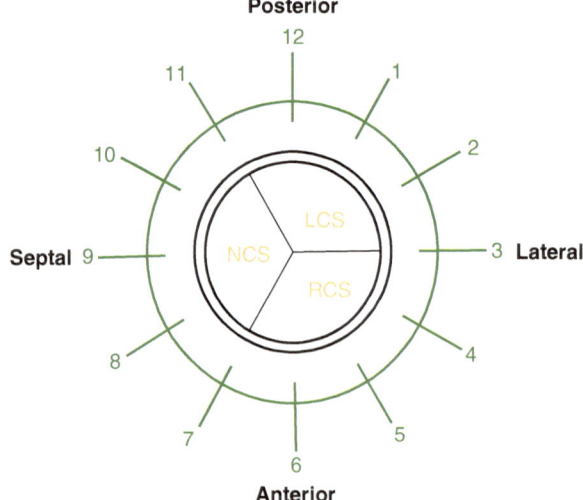

Fig. 2.9 Clockwise format from a surgeon's perspective of aortic valve. 3–4 o'clock is assigned to the commissure between the left and right coronary sinuses, 7–8 o'clock to the commissure between the right and non-coronary sinuses, and 11 o'clock to the commissure between the non-coronary and left coronary sinuses

Once aortic PVL has been identified and its precise localization is well-known, careful quantification using a multiparameter approach is strongly recommended. The process of grading aortic PVL should be comprehensive and integrative, using a combination of the qualitative and semiquantitative parameters [43–45].

2.4.2.1   Quantification of the Severity of Aortic PVL

Prosthetic Valve Structure
Initially, it is important to spend a few minutes on a detailed assessment of the prosthetic valve structure. A thorough visualization of the entire prosthesis, identifying the leaflets and prosthesis ring or stent is recommended. Rocking movement is usually associated with dehiscence and significant PLV. Other findings, such as endocarditis signs, can suggest the PVL aetiology.

Qualitative or Semiquantitative Parameters
Using TTE or TOE colour Doppler, the long-axis view is useful for measuring LVOT diameter and jet width. The ratios of regurgitant jet diameter to LVOT diameter from long-axis view and of jet area to LVOT area from short-axis view can be helpful to estimate the severity of aortic PVL. However, these parameters are highly influenced by the morphology and direction of regurgitant jet. Thus, in order to avoid underestimation, especially in regurgitant flows directed towards mitral anterior valve and LVOT wall, these parameters should be carefully assessed. A ratio of jet diameter to LVOT diameter greater than 25% has been associated with significant aortic PVL (Fig. 2.10).

Assessing the CW Doppler jet density of regurgitant flow may be helpful for a rough estimation of the severity. As an approximate guide, dense density suggests significant PVL, and incomplete or faint signal suggests trace or mild regurgitation.

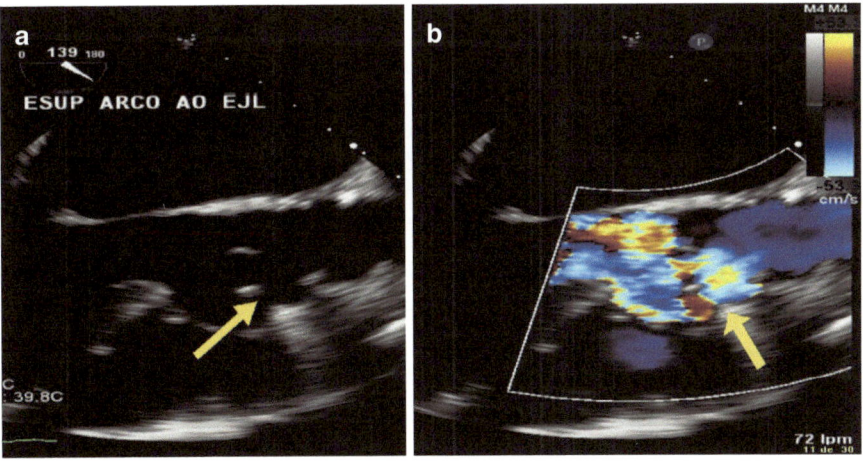

Fig. 2.10 TOE images with and without Colour Doppler of severe aortic PVL. (**a**) An echo dropout area outside the sewing ring can be visualized (*yellow arrow*) and then (**b**) confirmed by colour Doppler. In this case, an integrative approach for the assessment of the severity, combining quantitative and qualitative parameters should be required

Another parameter for grading severity is the pressure half-time. Values <200 ms suggest severe PVL, and values >500 ms almost completely rule out the presence of significant regurgitation. However, intermediate values of pressure half-time (200–500 ms) are less specific and may be influenced by other haemodynamic variables.

Prominent holodiastolic flow reversal in the ascending aorta (end-diastolic velocity greater than >18 cm/s) is associated with severe aortic PVL. Intermediate values should be integrated with additional parameters. Holodiastolic flow reversal in abdominal aorta is usually indicative of severe PVL.

Short-axis view at the level of the prosthesis sewing ring and more accurately 3D colour full volume allows the determination of the circumferential extent of paravalvular regurgitation. Values <10% of the sewing ring suggests mild, 10–20% suggests moderate and >20% suggests severe.

Quantitative Parameters
The width of the vena contracta, the narrowest part of the jet, is correlated with the severity of regurgitant jet, and it is a well-established parameter to assess the severity of native valve regurgitation. However, its application in PVL is commonly challenging because the prosthetic shadowing may obscure the regurgitant jet's origin and impede an accurate measure. This important limitation can be avoided by using colour Doppler 3D echocardiographic assessment that allows an accurate planimetry of the vena contracta area.

Other useful quantitative parameters are the measure of regurgitant volume and regurgitant fraction. These parameters can be calculated using the stroke volume and the mitral inflow volume. Similar values recommend for native aortic valve regurgitation assessing degree can be applied for aortic PVL.

Indirect Sign
Additional indirect signs are helpful in combination with quantitative and semi-quantitative parameters. Particularly, in the presence of aortic PVL, an increase in left ventricle end-diastolic and/or end-systolic diameters accompanied by an impairment of LVEF suggests a significant maintained volume overload and severe PVL.

It is important to note that it is essential to compare measurements with previous imaging examinations. However, sometimes it is difficult to separate postoperative abnormalities from new findings due to significant PVL (Table 2.2).

2.4.3   Paravalvular Regurgitation After Transcatheter Aortic Valve Replacement

Transcatheter aortic valve replacement (TAVR) has become a well-established treatment for appropriate patient with severe symptomatic aortic stenosis who is at high or intermediate risk for conventional open heart aortic valve surgery [71–73]. However, paravalvular aortic regurgitation (AR) after TAVR is common for both self-expanding and balloon-expandable prostheses, with an incidence that ranges between 45% and 93%, although most of them are trace or mild regurgitation and

Table 2.2 Echocardiographic criteria for severity evaluation of prosthetic aortic valve regurgitation

Aortic	Mild	Moderate	Severe
Valve structural parameters			
Mechanical or bioprosthesis	Usually normal	Usually abnormal	Usually abnormal
Qualitative or semiquantitative parameters			
Jet width in central jets (%LVOT diameter): colour Doppler	Narrow (<25)	Intermediate (25–65)	Large (>65)
Jet density: CW Doppler	Incomplete or faint	Dense	Dense
Jet deceleration rate (PHT, ms) CW Doppler	Slow (>500)	Variable (200–500)	Steep (<200)
LV outflow vs. RV outflow ratio: PW Doppler (ratio of stroke volumes or velocity-time integrals)	Slightly increased (>1.2)	Intermediate (>1.5)	Greatly increased (>1.8)
Diastolic flow reversal in the ascending aorta: PW Doppler	Absent or brief early diastolic	Intermediate	Prominent holodiastolic (end-diastolic velocity > 18 cm/s)
Diastolic flow reversal in the descending aorta: PW Doppler	Absent or brief early diastolic	Intermediate	Prominent, holodiastolic
Circumferential extent of paravalvular regurgitation (%)	<10	10–20	>20
Quantitative parameters			
Vena contracta width (mm)	<3	3–6	>6
Regurgitant volume (ml./beat)	<30	30–59	>60
Regurgitant fraction (%)	<30	30–49	>50
Indirect signs			
LV size	Normal	Normal/mildly dilated	Dilated

Adapted in part from Zoghbi WA, Chambers JB, Dumesnil JG, et al. Recommendations for evaluation of prosthetic valves with echocardiography and Doppler ultrasound. J Am Soc Echocardiogr 2009;22:975–1014

generally not progressive. Several studies have demonstrated that post-procedural significant AR is an independent predictor of mortality. Therefore, identification and accurate quantification is essential but is often challenging [74–77].

Although PVL assessment after TAVR follows mainly the same principles used for grading severity in other prosthetic valve aortic regurgitation, the exponential growing of this procedure and the well-known prognostic implications of AR after TAVR deserve a special dedication (Fig. 2.11).

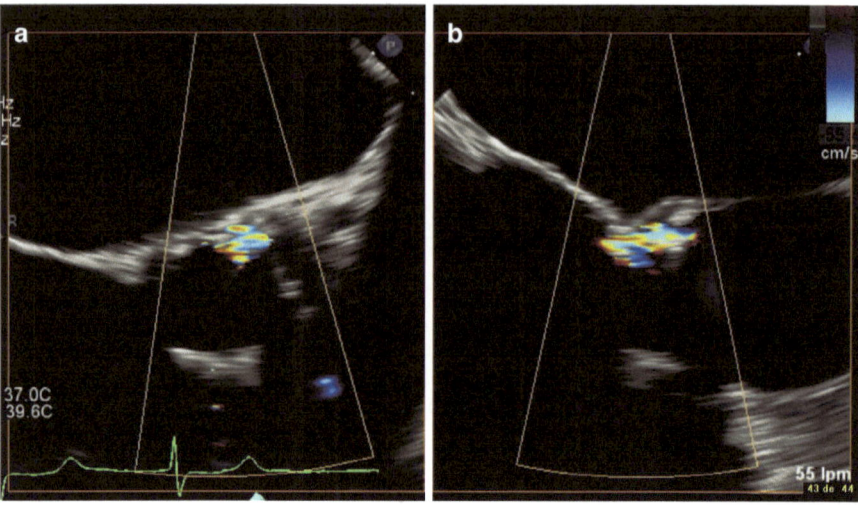

Fig. 2.11 Colour Doppler images of paravalvular aortic regurgitation after transcatheter aortic valve replacement. The yellow arrow indicate the regurgitation jet: (**a**) TOE short axis view and (**b**) TOE long axis view. The eccentric nature of PVL after TAVR and sometimes the presence of multiple regurgitant jets may lead to an over or underestimation of the severity

As with other PVLs, echocardiography is the gold standard imaging modality for identification and accurate assessment of AR after TAVR. TTE colour Doppler in parasternal short-axis and long-axis views may be helpful for identifying regurgitant jets. Whether AR is suspected using TTE, TOE examination is strongly recommended. The correct assessment of AR after TAVR should include evaluation of both paravalvular and central AR, with a combined measurement of whole aortic regurgitation (AR) reflecting the total regurgitation volume to LV. Frequently, 3D echocardiography provides better definition of size, number of jets and shape and allows a more accurate quantification of regurgitant severity [78–81].

Other imaging techniques, especially CMR, have been recognized as appropriate tools for AR assessment; although, further studies may provide validated data in order to recommend as routine clinical use.

The Valve Academic Research Consortium (VARC) consensus manuscript was published in January 2011 and updated in 2012 [82]. The aim of this document is to propose standardized consensus definitions for important endpoints in TAVR, including the assessment of AR. VARC-2 criteria for echocardiographic quantification of AR are detailed in Table 2.3.

2.4.4 Tricuspid Paravalvular Regurgitation

Although the same parameters of severity recommended for assessing severity of native tricuspid regurgitation can be used, there are limited data that support the applicability of them for evaluation of tricuspid PVL. Quantification parameters,

Table 2.3 Echocardiographic criteria for severity evaluation of transcatheter aortic valve regurgitation

TAVI	Mild	Moderate	Severe
Valve structural parameters			
Self-expanding or balloon expandable	Usually normal	Usually abnormal	Usually abnormal
Qualitative or semiquantitative parameters			
Jet width in central jets (%LVOT diameter): colour Doppler	Narrow (<25)	Intermediate (25–50)	Large (>50)
Jet density: CW Doppler	Incomplete or faint	Dense	Dense
Diastolic flow reversal in the descending aorta—PW	Absent or brief early diastolic	Intermediate	Prominent, holodiastolic
Circumferential extent of paravalvular regurgitation (%)	<10	10–29	>30
Quantitative parameters			
Regurgitant volume (mL/beat)	<30	30–59	≥60
Regurgitant fraction (%)	<30	30–49	≥50
EROA (cm^2)	0.10	0.10–0.29	≥0.30

Adapted in part from Kappetein AP, Head SJ, Genereux P, Piazza N, et al. Updated standardized endpoint definitions for transcatheter aortic valve implantation: the Valve Academic Research Consortium-2 consensus document. J Am Coll Cardiol. 2012; 60:1438–54

referential values and recommendations are mainly based on expert recommendation rather than on data from clinical studies.

TTE using colour Doppler may be useful for the screening of tricuspid PVL but is highly affected by the presence of acoustic shadowing, especially in mechanic prosthesis. For this reason, TOE assessment, with or without 3D full-volume colour images, is recommended in all patients for a detailed and accurate severity assessment. TOE examination should be focused on identifying the jet or jets as paravalvular or intravalvular.

Severity classification and haemodynamic significance are derived from the presence of congestive heart failure symptoms (characteristically right heart failure) combined with echocardiographic findings. The severity of tricuspid PVL can be assessed using semiquantitative parameters derived from components of the regurgitant flow, mainly jet density and jet area in the right atrium. A systolic flow reversal wave in hepatic venous flow has been related with severe tricuspid PVL. Although vena contracta width has not been widely validated for this purpose, values greater than 7 mm are associated with significant PVL.

Tricuspid PVL should be quantitated using an integrative echocardiographic approach. Table 2.4 summarizes the echocardiographic and Doppler parameters used in grading severity of prosthetic tricuspid valve regurgitation [43–45].

Table 2.4 Echocardiographic criteria for severity evaluation of prosthetic tricuspid valve regurgitation

Tricuspid	Mild	Moderate	Severe
Valve structural parameters			
Mechanical or bioprosthesis	Usually normal	Abnormal or valve dehiscence	Abnormal or valve dehiscence
Qualitative or semiquantitative parameters			
Jet area by colour Doppler (cm^2)	Mild (<5)	Intermediate (5–10)	Large (>10)
Jet density and contour: CW Doppler	Incomplete or faint, parabolic	Dense, variable contour	Dense with early peaking
Hepatic venous flow: PW Doppler	Systolic dominance	Systolic blunting	Systolic flow reversal
Circumferential extent of paravalvular regurgitation (%)	<10	10–20	>20
Quantitative parameters			
Vena contracta width (mm)	Not defined	Not defined, but <0.7	>0.7
Indirect signs			
Right atrium	Normal	Normal/mildly dilated	Dilated
Inferior vena cava	Normal	Normal/mildly dilated	Dilated
Right ventricle	Normal	Normal/mildly dilated	Dilated

Adapted in part from Zoghbi WA, Chambers JB, Dumesnil JG, et al. Recommendations for evaluation of prosthetic valves with echocardiography and Doppler ultrasound. J Am Soc Echocardiogr 2009;22:975–1014

2.4.5   Pulmonary Paravalvular Regurgitation

Grading the severity of pulmonary paravalvular regurgitation is usually complex, and there is limited data regarding echocardiographic assessment of prosthetic valves in the pulmonary position. For this reason and due to the paucity of well-validated parameters in prosthetic pulmonary valves, similar methods used in native pulmonary regurgitation can be used, and, sometimes, a subjective grading by experimented operator can be enough.

Basically, using colour Doppler, the severity of pulmonary PVL can be graded on the basis of the components of the jet, including regurgitant jet width, density of the regurgitant Doppler signal, vena contracta and its penetration depth into the RV outflow, in a similar manner to aortic PVL that is described previously. It is important to keep in mind that these semiquantitative parameters are highly influenced by the morphology and direction of the regurgitation flow and may underestimate the severity. In severe pulmonary PVL, a rapid equalization of right ventricle and pulmonary artery pressures can occur before the end of diastole. Other quantitative parameters, such as regurgitant volume and regurgitant fraction, can be measured from the difference between pulmonary and systemic flow.

Table 2.5 Echocardiographic criteria for severity evaluation of prosthetic pulmonary valve regurgitation

Pulmonary	Mild	Moderate	Severe
Valve structural parameters			
Mechanical or bioprosthesis	Usually normal	Abnormal or valve dehiscence	Abnormal or valve dehiscence
Qualitative or semiquantitative parameters			
Jet width in central jets (%RVOT diameter): colour Doppler	Narrow (<25)	Intermediate (25–50)	Large (>50)
Jet density: CW Doppler	Incomplete or faint	Dense	Dense
Jet deceleration rate by CW Doppler	Slow	Variable	Steep, early termination of diastolic flow
Pulmonary systolic flow vs. systemic flow by PW Doppler	Slightly increased	Intermediate	Greatly increased
Diastolic flow reversal in the pulmonary artery by PW Doppler	None	Present	Present
Circumferential extent of paravalvular regurgitation (%)	<10	10–20	>20
Indirect signs			
RV size	Normal	Normal/mildly dilated	Dilated

Adapted in part from Zoghbi WA, Chambers JB, Dumesnil JG, et al. Recommendations for evaluation of prosthetic valves with echocardiography and Doppler ultrasound. J Am Soc Echocardiogr 2009;22:975–1014

Table 2.5 summarizes the echocardiographic and Doppler parameters commonly used in grading severity of prosthetic pulmonary valve regurgitation [43–45].

2.5   Conclusion

Quantification parameters obtained by 2DTTE and 2DTOE can be used for the diagnosis and assessment of PVL, but often they are not enough for determining the precise morphology and anatomical shape. An accurate size, shape, origin and orientation evaluation of regurgitation jet is critical in determining the most appropriate treatment and, in case of percutaneous PVL closure, the most suitable device. 3D echocardiography has emerged in recent years as an indispensable imaging technique for detailed assessment of PVL and more accurate evaluation, and its use is recommended whenever possible. Therefore, a multimodality imaging approach, considering other imaging techniques such as cardiac CT and CMR, should be performed as routine clinical use for a comprehensive assessment, quantify severity and planning treatment of PVL.

References

1. Kliger C, Eiros R, Isasti G, Einhorn B, Jelnin V, Cohen H, et al. Review of surgical prosthetic paravalvular leaks: diagnosis and catheter-based closure. Eur Heart J. 2013;34(9):638–49.
2. Ionescu A, Fraser AG, Butchart EG. Prevalence and clinical significance of incidental para-prosthetic valvar regurgitation: a prospective study using transoesophageal echocardiography. Heart. 2003;89(11):1316–21.
3. Chen YT, Kan MN, Chen JS, Lin WW, Chang MK, WS H, et al. Detection of prosthetic mitral valve leak: a comparative study using transesophageal echocardiography, transthoracic echo-cardiography, and auscultation. J Clin Ultrasound. 1990;18(7):557–61.
4. Bernal JM, Rabasa JM, Cagigas JC, Echevarria JR, Carrion MF, Revuelta JM. Valve-related complications with the Hancock I porcine bioprosthesis. A twelve- to fourteen-year follow-up study. J Thorac Cardiovasc Surg. 1991;101(5):871–80.
5. Miller DL, Morris JJ, Schaff HV, Mullany CJ, Nishimura RA, Orszulak TA. Reoperation for aortic valve periprosthetic leakage: identification of patients at risk and results of operation. J Heart Valve Dis. 1995;4(2):160–5.
6. Jindani A, Neville EM, Venn G, Williams BT. Paraprosthetic leak: a complication of cardiac valve replacement. J Cardiovasc Surg. 1991;32(4):503–8.
7. Wasowicz M, Meineri M, Djalani G, et al. Early complications and immediate postoperative outcomes of paravalvular leaks after valve replacement surgery. J Cardiothorac Vasc Anesth. 2011;25(4):610–4.
8. Rallidis LS, Moyssakis IE, Ikonomidis I, Nihoyannopoulos P. Natural history of early aortic paraprosthetic regurgitation: a five-year follow-up. Am Heart J. 1999;138:351–7.
9. De Cicco G, Lorusso R, Colli A, Nicolini F, Fragnito C, Grimaldi T, et al. Aortic valve peripros-thetic leakage: anatomic observations and surgical results. Ann Thorac Surg. 2005;79:1480–5.
10. De Cicco G, Russo C, Moreo A, Beghi C, Fucci C, Gerometta P, et al. Mitral valve peri-prosthetic leakage: anatomical observations in 135 patients from a multicentre study. Eur J Cardiothorac Surg. 2006;30:887–91.
11. Safi AM, Kwan T, Afflu E, et al. Paravalvular regurgitation: a rare complication following valve replacement surgery. Angiology. 2000;51:479–87.
12. Pate GE, Al Zubaidi A, Chandavimol M, Thompson CR, Munt BI, Webb JG. Percutaneous closure of prosthetic paravalvular leaks: case series and review. Catheter Cardiovasc Interv. 2006;68:528–33.
13. Davila-Roman VG, Waggoner AD, Kennard ED, Holubkov R, Jamieson WR, Englberger L, et al. Prevalence and severity of paravalvular regurgitation in the artificial valve endocarditis reduction trial (avert) echocardiography study. J Am Coll Cardiol. 2004;44:1467–72.
14. García E, Sandoval J, Unzue L, et al. Paravalvular leaks: mechanisms, diagnosis and manage-ment. EuroIntervention. 2012;8(Suppl Q):Q41–52.
15. Ruiz CE, Jelnin V, Kronzon I, Dudiy Y, Del Valle-Fernandez R, Einhorn BN, et al. Clinical outcomes in patients undergoing percutaneous closure of periprosthetic paravalvular leaks. J Am Coll Cardiol. 2011;58:2210–7.
16. Sorajja P, Cabalka AK, Hagler DJ, Rihal CS. Percutaneous repair of paravalvular prosthetic regurgitation: acute and 30-day outcomes in 115 patients. Circ Cardiovasc Interv. 2011;4:314–21.
17. Skoularigis J, Essop MR, Skudicky D, Middlemost SJ, Sareli P. Frequency and severity of intravascular hemolysis after left-sided cardiac valve replacement with medtronic hall and St. Jude medical prostheses, and influence of prosthetic type, position, size and number. Am J Cardiol. 1993;71:587–91.
18. Hourihan M, Perry SB, Mandell VS, Keane JF, Rome JJ, Bittl JA, et al. Transcatheter umbrella closure of valvular and paravalvular leaks. J Am Coll Cardiol. 1992;20:1371–7.
19. Dumesnil J, Pibarot P. Doppler echocardiographic evaluation of prosthetic valve function. Heart. 2012;98:69–78.
20. Zoghbi WA, Enriquez-Sarano M, Foster E, et al. Recommendations for evaluation of the sever-ity of native valvular regurgitation with two-dimensional and Doppler echocardiography. J Am Soc Echocardiogr. 2003;16:777–802.

21. Effron MK, Popp RL. Two-dimensional echocardiographic assessment of bioprosthetic valve dysfunction and infective endocarditis. J Am Coll Cardiol. 1983;2:597–606.
22. Daniel LB, Grigg LE, Weisel RD, Rakowski H. Comparison of transthoracic and transesophageal assessment of prosthetic valve dysfunction. Echocardiography. 1990;7:83–95.
23. Alton M, Pasierski TJ, Orsinelli DA, Eaton GM, Pearson AC. Comparison of transthoracic and transesophageal echocardiography in evaluation of 47 Starr-Edwards prosthetic valves. J Am Coll Cardiol. 1992;20:1503–11.
24. Van den Brink RB. Evaluation of prosthetic heart valves by transesophageal echocardiography: problems, pitfalls, and timing of echocardiography. Semin Cardiothorac Vasc Anesth. 2006;10(1):89–100.
25. Rahko PS. Assessing prosthetic mitral valve regurgitation by transoesophageal echo/Doppler. Heart. 2004;90(5):476–8.
26. Bach DS. Transesophageal echocardiographic (TEE) evaluation of prosthetic valves. Cardiol Clin. 2000;18:751–71.
27. Vitarelli A, Conde Y, Cimino E, et al. Assessment of severity of mechanical prosthetic mitral regurgitation by transoesophageal echocardiography. Heart. 2004;90:539–44.
28. Flachskampf FA, Hoffmann R, Franke A, et al. Does multiplane transesophageal echocardiography improve the assessment of prosthetic valve regurgitation? J Am Soc Echocardiogr. 1995;8:70–8.
29. Tsang W, Weinert L, Kronzon I, Lang RM. Three-dimensional echocardiography in the assessment of prosthetic valves. Rev Esp Cardiol. 2011;64:1–7.
30. Kort S. Real-time 3-dimensional echocardiography for prosthetic valve endocarditis: initial experience. J Am Soc Echocardiogr. 2006;19:130–9.
31. Sugeng L, Shernan SK, Weinert L, et al. Real-time three-dimensional transesophageal echocardiography in valve disease: comparison with surgical findings and evaluation of prosthetic valves. J Am Soc Echocardiogr. 2008;21:1347–54.
32. Singh P, Manda J, Hsiung MC, et al. Live/real time three-dimensional transesophageal echocardiographic evaluation of mitral and aortic valve prosthetic paravalvular regurgitation. Echocardiography. 2009;26:980–7.
33. Kronzon I, Sugeng L, Perk G, et al. Real-time 3-dimensional transesophageal echocardiography in the evaluation of post-operative mitral annuloplasty ring and prosthetic valve dehiscence. J Am Coll Cardiol. 2009;53:1543–7.
34. Marcos-Alberca P, Zamorano JL, Sanchez T, et al. Intraoperative monitoring with transesophageal real-time three-dimensional echocardiography during transapical prosthetic aortic valve implantation. Rev Esp Cardiol. 2010;63:352–6.
35. Dobarro D, Gomez-Rubin MC, Lopez-Fernandez T, et al. Real time three-dimensional transesophageal echocardiography for guiding percutaneous mitral valvuloplasty. Echocardiography. 2009;26:746–8.
36. Perk G, Lang RM, Garcia-Fernandez MA, et al. Use of real time three-dimensional transesophageal echocardiography in intracardiac catheter based interventions. J Am Soc Echocardiogr. 2009;22:865–82.
37. Becerra JM, Almeria C, de Isla LP, Zamorano J. Usefulness of 3D transoesophageal echocardiography for guiding wires and closure devices in mitral perivalvular leaks. Eur J Echocardiogr. 2009;10(8):979–81.
38. Osman F, Steeds R. Use of intra-cardiac ultrasound in the diagnosis of prosthetic valve malfunction. Eur J Echocardiogr. 2007;8:392–4.
39. Asrress KN, Mitchell AR. Intracardiac echocardiography. Heart. 2009;95:327–31.
40. Deftereos S, Giannopoulos G, Raisakis K, Kaoukis A, Kossyvakis C. Intracardiac echocardiography imaging of periprosthetic valvular regurgitation. Eur J Echocardiogr. 2010;11(5):E20.
41. Bartel T, Konorza T, Neudorf U, Ebralize T, Eggebrecht H, Gutersohn A, et al. Intra4cardiac echocardiography: an ideal guiding tool for device closure of interatrial communications. Eur J Echocardiogr. 2005;6:92–6.
42. Picano E, Pibarot P, Lancellotti P, et al. The emerging role of exercise testing and stress echocardiography in valvular heart disease. J Am Coll Cardiol. 2009;54:2251–60.

43. Lancellotti P, Pibarot P, Chambers J, Edvardsen T, Delgado V, Dulgheru R, et al. Recommendations for the imaging assessment of prosthetic heart valves: a report from the European Association of Cardiovascular Imaging endorsed by the Chinese Society of Echocardiography, the Inter-American Society of Echocardiography, and the Brazilian Department of Cardiovascular Imaging. Eur Heart J Cardiovasc Imaging. 2016;17(6):589–90.

44. Zoghbi WA, Chambers JB, Dumesnil JG, Foster E, Gottdiener JS, Grayburn PA, et al. Recommendations for evaluation of prosthetic valves with echocardiography and Doppler ultrasound: a report From the American Society of Echocardiography's Guidelines and Standards Committee and the Task Force on Prosthetic Valves, developed in conjunction with the American College of Cardiology Cardiovascular Imaging Committee, Cardiac Imaging Committee of the American Heart Association, the European Association of Echocardiography, a registered branch of the European Society of Cardiology, the Japanese Society of Echocardiography and the Canadian Society of Echocardiography, endorsed by the American College of Cardiology Foundation, American Heart Association, European Association of Echocardiography, a registered branch of the European Society of Cardiology, the Japanese Society of Echocardiography, and Canadian Society of Echocardiography. J Am Soc Echocardiogr. 2009;22(9):975–1014. quiz 82–4

45. Nishimura RA, Otto CM, Bonow RO, Carabello BA, Erwin JP III, Guyton RA, et al. AHA/ACC guideline for the management of patients with valvular heart disease: a report of the American College of Cardiology/American Heart Association Task Force on Practice Guidelines. J Am Coll Cardiol. 2014;63(22):e57–185.

46. Magne J, Lancellotti P, Pierard LA. Exercise pulmonary hypertension in asymptomatic degenerative mitral regurgitation. Circulation. 2010;122:33–41.

47. Jaffe WM, Coverdale HA, Roche AHG, et al. Rest and exercise hemodynamics of 20 to 23 mm allograft, Medtronic Intact (porcine), and St. Jude medical valves in the aortic position. J Thorac Cardiovasc Surg. 1990;100:167–74.

48. Lancellotti P, Magne J. Stress echocardiography in regurgitant valve disease. Circ Cardiovasc Imaging. 2013;6(5):840–9.

49. Pibarot P, Dumesnil JG, Jobin J, et al. Usefulness of the indexed effective orifice area at rest in predicting an increase in gradient during maximum exercise in patients with a bioprosthesis in the aortic valve position. Am J Cardiol. 1999;83:542–6.

50. Chambers J, Rimington H, Rajani R, et al. Hemodynamic performance on exercise: comparison of a stentless and stented biological aortic valve replacement. J Heart Valve Dis. 2004;13:729–33.

51. Newland JA, Tamuno P, Pasupati S, et al. Emerging role of MDCT in planning complex structural transcatheter intervention. J Am Coll Cardiol Imag. 2014;7:627–31.

52. Raff GL, Abidov A, Achenbach S, et al. Society of Cardiovascular Computed Tomography. SCCT guidelines for the interpretation and reporting of coronary computed tomographic angiography. J Cardiovasc Comput Tomogr. 2009;3:122–36.

53. Blanke P, Schoepf UJ, Leipsic JA. Computed tomography in transcatheter aortic valve replacement. Radiology. 2013;269:650–69.

54. Leipsic J, LaBounty TM, Ajlan AM, et al. A prospective randomized trial comparing image quality, study interpretability, and radiation dose of narrow acquisition window with widened acquisition window protocols in prospectively ECG-triggered coronary computed tomography angiography. J Cardiovasc Comput Tomogr. 2013;7:18–24.

55. Jelnin V, Co J, Muneer B, Swaminathan B, Toska S, Ruiz CE. Three dimensional CT angiography for patients with congenital heart disease: Scanning protocol for pediatric patients. Catheter Cardiovasc Interv. 2006;67:120–6.

56. Quail MA, Nordmeyer J, Schievano S, Reinthaler M, Mullen MJ, Taylor AM. Use of cardiovascular magnetic resonance imaging for TAVR assessment in patients with bioprosthetic aortic valves: comparison with computed tomography. Eur J Radiol. 2012;81:3912–7.

57. Numata S, Tsutsumi Y, Monta O, Yamazaki S, Seo H, Yoshida S, et al. Mechanical valve evaluation with four-dimensional computed tomography. J Heart Valve Dis. 2013;22:837–42.

58. O'Neill AC, Martos R, Murtagh G, Ryan ER, McCreery C, Keane D, et al. Practical tips and tricks for assessing prosthetic valves and detecting paravalvular regurgitation using cardiac CT. J Cardiovasc Comput Tomogr. 2014;8(4):323–7.
59. Soulen RL, Budinger TF, Higgins CB. Magnetic resonance imaging of prosthetic heart valves. Radiology. 1985;154:705–7.
60. Walker PG, Pedersen EM, Oyre S, Flepp L, Ringgaard S, Heinrich RS, et al. Magnetic resonance velocity imaging: A new method for prosthetic heart valve study. J Heart Valve Dis. 1995;4:296–307.
61. Salaun E, Jacquier A, Theron A, Giorgi R, Lambert M, Jaussaud N, et al. Value of CMR in quantification of paravalvular aortic regurgitation after TAVI. Eur Heart J Cardiovasc Imaging. 2016;17(1):41–50.
62. Lerakis S, Hayek S, Arepalli CD, Thourani V, Babaliaros V. Cardiac magnetic resonance for paravalvular leaks in post-transcatheter aortic valve replacement. Circulation. 2014;129:e430–1.
63. Ribeiro HB, Le Ven F, Larose E, Dahou A, Nombela-Franco L, Urena M, et al. Cardiac magnetic resonance versus transthoracic echocardiography for the assessment and quantification of aortic regurgitation in patients undergoing transcatheter aortic valve implantation. Heart. 2014;100:1924–32.
64. Hartlage GR, Babaliaros VC, Thourani VH, Hayek S, Chrysohoou C, Ghasemzadeh N, et al. The role of cardiovascular magnetic resonance in stratifying paravalvular leak severity after transcatheter aortic valve replacement: an observational outcome study. J Cardiovasc Magn Reson. 2014;16:93.
65. Hundley WG, Bluemke DA, Finn JP, Flamm SD, Fogel MA, Friedrich MG, et al. ACCF/ACR/AHA/NASCI/SCMR 2010 expert consensus document on cardiovascular magnetic resonance: a report of the American College of Cardiology Foundation Task Force on Expert Consensus Documents. Circulation. 2010;121:2462–508.
66. Myerson SG, D'Arcy J, Mohiaddin R, Greenwood JP, Karamitsos TD, Francis JM, et al. Aortic regurgitation quantification using cardiovascular magnetic resonance: association with clinical outcome. Circulation. 2012;126:1452–60.
67. Gelfand EV, Hughes S, Hauser TH, Yeon SB, Goepfert L, Kissinger KV, et al. Severity of mitral and aortic regurgitation as assessed by cardiovascular magnetic resonance: optimizing correlation with Doppler echocardiography. J Cardiovasc Magn Reson. 2006;8:503–7.
68. Cawley PJ, Hamilton-Craig C, Owens DS, Krieger EV, Strugnell WE, Mitsumori L, et al. Prospective comparison of valve regurgitation quantitation by cardiac magnetic resonance imaging and transthoracic echocardiography. Circ Cardiovasc Imaging. 2013;6:48–57.66.
69. Franco E, Almeria C, de Agustin JA, Arreo Del Val V, Gomez de Diego JJ, Garcia Fernandez MA, et al. Three-dimensional color Doppler transesophageal echocardiography for mitral paravalvular leak quantification and evaluation of percutaneous closure success. J Am Soc Echocardiogr. 2014;27(11):1153–63.
70. Arribas-Jimenez A, Rama-Merchan JC, Barreiro-Perez M, Merchan-Gomez S, Iscar-Galan A, Martin-Garcia A, et al. Utility of real-time 3-dimensional transesophageal echocardiography in the assessment of mitral paravalvular leak. Circ J. 2016;80(3):738–44.
71. Leon MB, Smith CR, Mack M, et al. Transcatheter aortic-valve implantation for aortic stenosis in patients who cannot undergo surgery. N Engl J Med. 2010;363(17):1597–607.
72. Smith CR, Leon MB, Mack MJ, et al. Transcatheter versus surgical aortic-valve replacement in high-risk patients. N Engl J Med. 2011;364(23):2187–98.
73. Hahn RT, Pibarot P, Stewart WJ, et al. Comparison of transcatheter and surgical aortic valve replacement in severe aortic stenosis: a longitudinal study of echocardiography parameters in cohort A of the PARTNER trial (Placement of Aortic Transcatheter Valves). J Am Coll Cardiol. 2013;61(25):2514–21.
74. Kodali SK, Williams MR, Smith CR, Svensson LG, Webb JG, Makkar RR, et al. PARTNER Trial Investigators. Two-year outcomes after transcatheter or surgical aortic-valve replacement. N Engl J Med. 2012;366:1686–95.

75. Rodés-Cabau J, Webb JG, Cheung A, Ye J, Dumont E, Osten M, et al. Long-term outcomes after transcatheter aortic valve implantation. Insights on prognostic factors and valve durability from the Canadian multicenter experience. J Am Coll Cardiol. 2012;60:1864–75.
76. Makkar RR, Fontana GP, Jilaihawi H, Kapadia S, Pichard AD, Douglas PS, et al. Transcatheter aortic-valve replacement for inoperable severe aortic stenosis. N Engl J Med. 2012;366:1696–704.
77. Athappan G, Patvardhan E, Tuzcu EM, Svensson LG, Lemos PA, Fraccaro C, et al. Incidence, predictors, and outcomes of aortic regurgitation after transcatheter aortic valve replacement: meta-analysis and systematic review of literature. J Am Coll Cardiol. 2013;61:1585–95.
78. Zamorano JL, Badano LP, Bruce C, Chan KL, Gonçalves A, Hahn RT, et al. EAE/ASE recommendations for the use of echocardiography in new transcatheter interventions for valvular heart disease. J Am Soc Echocardiogr. 2011;24:937–65.
79. Genereux P, Head SJ, Hahn R, Daneault B, Kodali S, Williams MR, et al. Paravalvular leak after transcatheter aortic valve replacement: the new Achilles' heel? A comprehensive review of the literature. J Am Coll Cardiol. 2013;61:1125–36.
80. Sinning JM, Vasa-Nicotera M, Chin D, Hammerstingl C, Ghanem A, Bence J, et al. Evaluation and management of paravalvular aortic regurgitation after transcatheter aortic valve replacement. J Am Coll Cardiol. 2013;62:11–20.
81. Gonçalves A, Almeria C, Marcos-Alberca P, Feltes G, Hernández-Antolín R, Rodriguez E, et al. Three-dimensional echocardiography in paravalvular aortic regurgitation assessment after transcatheter aortic valve implantation. J Am Soc Echocardiogr. 2012;25:47–55.
82. Kappetein AP, Head SJ, Genereux P, Piazza N, van Mieghem NM, Blackstone EH, et al. Updated standardized endpoint definitions for transcatheter aortic valve implantation: the Valve Academic Research Consortium-2 consensus document. J Am Coll Cardiol. 2012;60:1438–54.
83. Lesser JR, Han BK, Newell M, Schwartz RS, Pedersen W, Sorajja P. Use of cardiac CT angiography to assist in the diagnosis and treatment of aortic prosthetic paravalvular leak: a practical guide. J Cardiovasc Comput Tomogr. 2015;9(3):159–64.

Chapter 3
Transcatheter Paravalvular Leak Closure: History, Available Devices

I. Cruz-Gonzalez[†], C.E. Ruiz, Z.M. Hijazi, and J.C. Rama-Merchan[†]

3.1 Introduction: First Transcatheter Procedures

The incidence of paravalvular leaks (PVLs) after surgical valve replacement is estimated to be 2–17% [1–3]. If symptomatic or if the severity of the PVL is moderate or severe, redo surgery is a therapeutic option, but this is accompanied by a high perioperative risk and a high recurrence rate [2–4].

Percutaneous closure of PVL has been increasingly performed in the last few years with a success rate (successful deployment of an occlusive device across the paravalvular leak without any mechanical interference with the valve prosthesis, or acute conversion to surgery) reported to be around 80% [5–10]. Most of the devices used today have not been designed, tested, or approved for PVL closure, and they are used "off-label" for this purpose. PVLs are variable in size and shape with many being crescentic and serpiginous, not cylindrical which makes it extremely difficult for one device to fit in all PVLs [11–13].

The first successful percutaneous closure of PVLs was reported by Hourihan and colleagues in 1992 with the use of the Rashkind double-umbrella device [14]. Initially this device was intended for closure of patent ductus arteriosus (PDA), collateral channels, aortopulmonary windows, and venous connections [15–17]. Its modification (clamshell device) was successfully used for closure of a variety of

†I. Cruz-Gonzalez and J. C. Rama-Merchan contributed equally to this work.

I. Cruz-Gonzalez, M.D., Ph.D. (✉) • J.C. Rama-Merchan, M.D., Ph.D.
University Hospital of Salamanca, Universtiy of Salamanca, Salamanca, Spain
e-mail: cruzgonzalez.ignacio@gmail.com

C.E. Ruiz, M.D., Ph.D.
The Joseph M. Sanzari Children's Hospital, Hackensack UMC Heart and Vascular Hospital, Hackensack, NJ, USA

Z.M. Hijazi, M.D.
Weill Cornell Medicine, Sidra Cardiovascular Center of Excellence, Doha, Qatar

© Springer Nature Singapore Pte Ltd. 2017
G. Smolka et al. (eds.), *Transcatheter Paravalvular Leak Closure*,
DOI 10.1007/978-981-10-5400-6_3

septal defects [16, 18, 19]. Early attempts to close PVL were also made using Gianturco coils [20, 21]. Nevertheless, none of these devices fulfilled the requirements for an ideal PVL closure device.

The ideal PVL closure device should have the following criteria: (a) conform to the often "irregular" defects, (b) have low-profile deliverability, (c) be repositionable and retrievable, (d) avoid interference with prosthetic valve leaflets, (e) accomplish complete closure of the defect, (f) have low risk of embolization or dislodgement, and (h) should not be thrombogenic.

This chapter will focus on the currently available devices for PVL closure.

3.2   Devices Presently Used for Transcatheter PVL Closure

Today, most PVL closure procedures are performed with the off-label use of Amplatzer devices [5, 8, 10, 22, 23] (St. Jude Medical, St. Paul, MN, USA; Fig. 3.1). These devices are either cylindrical (Amplatzer septal occluder (ASO), Amplatzer muscular VSD occluder (AmVSDo), Amplatzer duct occluder (ADO), Amplatzer vascular plug (AVP) II and IV) or oblong shaped (AVP III). Although all of these devices may be suitable in some or even most of the cases, they clearly have several limitations including the sizes available, shape, and delivery system features.

In addition, to date, no specific device has been approved by the US Food and Drug Administration (FDA) for the indication of percutaneous PVL closure. Therefore, therapeutic options are limited to "off-label" use. The AVP II is the device most commonly used in the USA to close PVLs; however, the AVP III is the most frequently used outside of the USA [10, 22, 24]. Currently, the only device specifically approved for PVL closure by the European Commission (EC) is the Occlutech paravalvular leak device (PLD) (Occlutech, Helsingborg, Sweden) [25].

3.3   Amplatzer™ Family of Vascular Plugs

3.3.1   Amplatzer Vascular Plug II

The AVP II is a self-expandable nitinol mesh occlusion device (Figs. 3.1d and 3.3c, d). It has three segments, including the central lobe, and two discs on each side of the lobe. Because of its tri-lobar design, AVP II has six layers of mesh, giving the device better occlusive properties. It is available in diameters ranging from 3 mm to 22 mm. The device comes preloaded and has a proximal microscrew to permit the attachment to a delivery cable. It can be implanted through a 4 Fr long sheath for 3–8 mm devices, through a 5 Fr long sheath for 10 and 12 mm devices, through a 6 Fr sheath for 14 and 16 mm devices and through a 7 Fr long sheath for larger devices (Table 3.1).

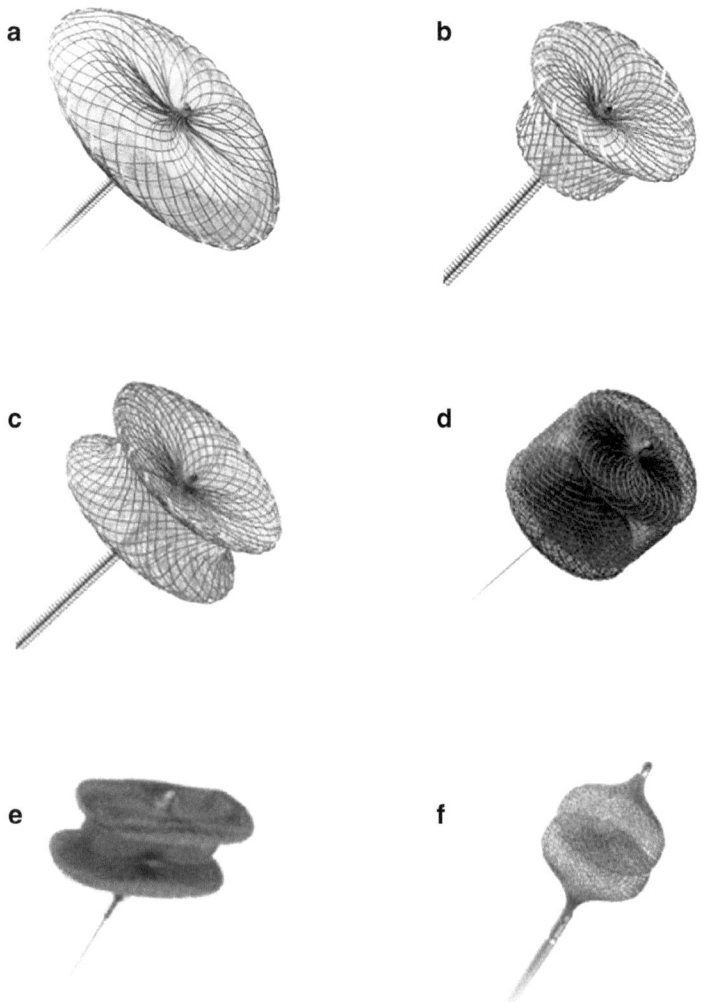

Fig. 3.1 Amplatzer devices. (**a**) Amplatzer septal occluder device, (**b**) Amplatzer duct occluder device, (**c**) Amplatzer muscular VSD occluder device, (**d**) Amplatzer vascular plug II device, (**e**) Amplatzer vascular plug III device, (**f**) Amplatzer vascular plug IV device

Sorajja et al. [26] reported a retrospective review of 126 patients undergoing percutaneous PVL closure. The AVP II was the device most used. Technical and procedure success were 91 and 76%, respectively. The 3-year estimate for survival was 64.3% (95% confidence interval, 52.1–76.8%). Among survivors, 72% of patients who had presented with heart failure were free of severe symptoms and

Table 3.1 Amplatzer devices: main characteristics

	Size (central waist)	Length (central waist)	Difference between disc and central waist	Sheath size (Fr)	Comments
ASO	4–40 mm (every 1 mm up to 20 mm, >20 mm, every 2 mm)	3–4 mm	8–12 mm (ASO 4–10) 10/14 mm (ASO >11) 10/16 mm (ASO >34)	6–12	
AmVSDo	4–18 mm (every 2 mm)	7 mm	8 mm	5–9	– Useful to close large PVLs – Risk of interference with mechanical leaflets
ADO	5–16 mm distal end and 4–14 mm proximal	5–8 mm	4 mm (ADO 5/4–8/6) 6 mm (ADO 10/8–16/14)	5–7	
AVP II	3–22 mm (every 2 mm)	6 mm	–	4–7	– Useful to close long tunnel-shaped PVLs with a large central cavity
AVP III	Long axis: 4–14 mm Short axis: 2–5 mm	2–5 mm	2 mm	4–7	– Useful to close crescent shaped PVLs
AVP IV	4–8 mm	10–13.5 mm	–	4–5	– Can be deployed through a 4 Fr diagnostic catheter – Often used in PVL closure after TAVI

ASO Amplatzer septal occluder, AmVSDo Amplatzer muscular VSD occluder, ADO Amplatzer duct occluder, AVP Amplatzer vascular plug, PVL paravalvular leak

need for cardiac surgery. For those with no, mild, or moderate or severe residual regurgitation, 3-year estimate of survival free of death or need for surgery was 63.3%, 58.3%, and 30.3% ($p = 0.01$), respectively.

Also, Ruiz et al. [8] reported a series of 43 patients (57 percutaneous PVLs) undergoing percutaneous PVL closure. The ADO device was used in 68.9% of the procedures, the AmVSDo (Amplatzer muscular VSD occluder) device in 18.7%, the AVP II device in 8.3%, and the ASO (Amplatzer septal occluder) device in 4.1%. Closure was successful (deployment of an occlusive device across the paravalvular leak without any mechanical interference with the valve prosthesis) in 86% of defects, and clinical success was achieved in 86% of the patients in whom procedure was successful. The survival rates for patients at 6, 12, and 18 months after PVL closures were 91.9%, 89.2%, and 86.5%, respectively.

3.3.2 Amplatzer Vascular Plug III

The AVP III is a nitinol-based device with an elliptical lobe that adapts to the often crescent-shaped defects. The lobe is covered by two discs on each side protruding from the lobe by only 2 mm, in order to reduce the risk of interference with mechanical valve leaflets (Figs. 3.1e and 3.3a, b). Different sizes from 4 × 2 mm to 14 × 5 mm are available, fitting through a 4–7 Fr sheath (Table 3.1). The AVP III device sizing requires careful examination of the PVL anatomy, specifically, the diameter and length of the defect, and its relationship to the surrounding cardiac structures. This device received the EC Mark in 2008 for vascular occlusion. It does not have FDA approval.

Nietlispach et al. [9] first reported feasibility, safety, and efficacy of AVP III for PVL closure. In this study, five patients with severe paravalvular mitral and aortic regurgitation underwent PVL closure. Implantation of the device was successfully accomplished in all. There was no procedural mortality. At a median follow-up of 191 days (interquartile range [IQR] 169–203 days), all patients were alive. Also, patients have shown significant improvement in NYHA functional class, hemoglobin and creatinine levels. Median echocardiographic follow-up at 58 days (IQR 56–70 days) reported residual regurgitation to be reduced from grade 4 to grade 2 (IQR 1.5–2.25).

Cruz-Gonzalez et al. [10] reported a series of 33 patients (34 PVLs, 27 mitral and 7 aortic) undergoing percutaneous PVL closure using also the AVP III. The device was successfully implanted in 94% of patients, and successful closure (defined as regurgitation reduction ≥1 grade) was achieved in 91% of patients. There were no procedure-related deaths, myocardial infarctions, or stroke. At 90 days, survival was 100%, and more than 90% showed significant clinical improvement. Also, Sanchez-Recalde et al. [22] reported a series of 20 patients with PVLs. Closure was attempted for 23 PVLs (17 mitral and 6 aortic). The AVP III device was used in 18 patients (86%). Implantation was successful in 87% of the defects, and the procedure was successful in 83% (with success being defined as a reduction in regurgitation of ≥1 degree). Survival at 1 year was 64.7% and survival free of the composite event of death/surgery was 58.8%. Survivors showed significant improvement in functional class.

3.3.3 Amplatzer Vascular Plug IV

The AVP IV is a double-lobed occluder device (Figs. 3.1f and 3.3e, f). It has four layers of occluding mesh. The main advantage of this device is the flexibility and small profile. The AVP IV is available in a range of diameters from 4 to 8 mm (Table 3.1). It can be delivered through a 0.038-inch diagnostic catheter lumen and placed in very serpiginous and long tunnel PVLs, such as those that occur after transcatheter aortic valve replacement (TAVR) [27, 28]. Saia et al. [27] recently reported a series of 24 patients (27 procedures) with significant aortic paravalvular regurgitation (PVR) after TAVR underwent percutaneous PVL closure. The most frequently used device was AVP (II, III and IV) in 80% of the cases. Overall, 88.9% (24 of 27) of the procedures were technically successful, and the results assessed by echocardiography were durable. Also, Cruz-Gonzalez et al. have reported a case of severe aortic PVR after TAVR successfully closed using simultaneously AVP III and IV devices [28].

The AVP IV device can be deployed, recaptured and redeployed to assist secure placement. This device received the EC Mark and FDA approval for vascular occlusion.

3.4   Occlutech PVL Device

The Occlutech PLD is a double-disc device made of nitinol braided mesh with a wire range of 67–107 μm according to the device size. This device obtained the EC Mark approval for this use in 2014.

The device is available in two different shapes, square and rectangular, and two different connections between the discs, waist and twist (Figs. 3.2 and 3.3c, d). Both the rectangular and square designs have 35% more surface areas compared to a circular design, which increases the area covered by one device. Also, the two discs

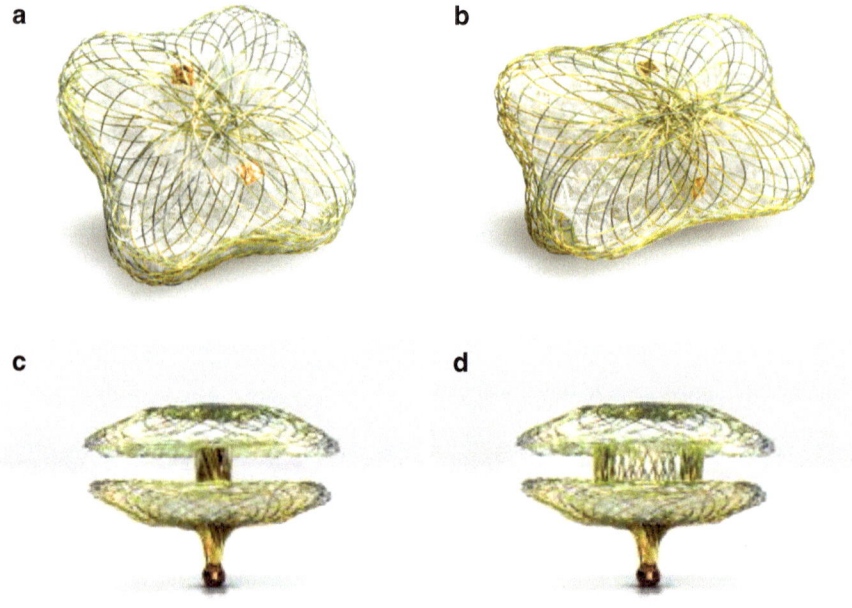

Fig. 3.2 Occlutech paravalvular leak device. Square-shaped (**a**) and rectangular-shaped (**b**) designs. Twist (**c**) and waist (**d**) connections

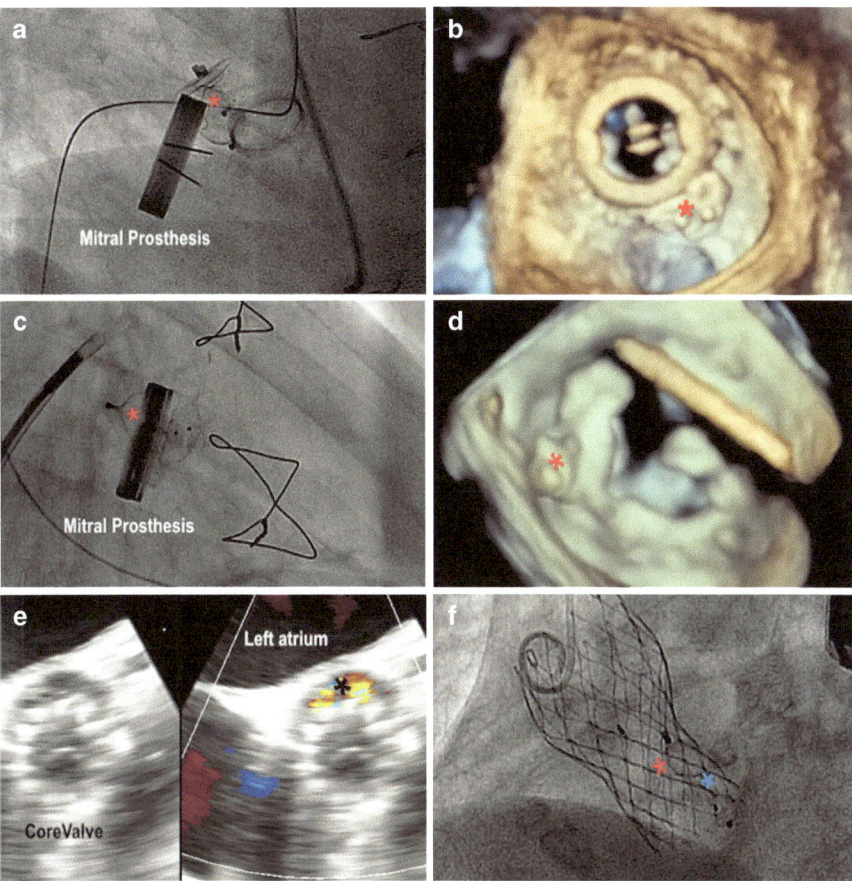

Fig. 3.3 Paravalvular leaks closure devices: angiographic and echocardiography images. (**a, b**) Mitral PVL successfully closed using two AVP III devices (*red asterisk*), (**c, d**) mitral PVL successfully closed using an Occlutech device (*red asterisk*), (**e, f**) posterior aortic PVL after TAVR (*black asterisk*) successfully closed using AVP III (*blue asterisk*) and AVP IV (*red asterisk*) devices

are attached with a twist bundle of wires to suit the defect anatomy and to eliminate the risk of defect enlargement [29].

The Occlutech PLD is available in different sizes ranging from 3 to 7 mm with a circular waist for the square device that requires 5–7 Fr sheaths and from 4 × 2 to 12 × 5 mm with an ellipsoid waist for the rectangular device that requires 5–8 Fr sheaths for delivery (Table 3.2) [29]. There are two gold radiopaque markers to indicate the disc frame position and the largest part of the elliptical waist. This provides the implanting physician accuracy in positioning the device correctly in the defect as seen by fluoroscopy. The device can be delivered from both transapical and transfemoral access using small delivery catheters.

Table 3.2 Occlutech paravalvular leak devices: main characteristics

	Length of the distal disc	Length of the proximal disc	Length × width	Diameter of the waist for square PLD	Defect size	Size (Fr)
Occlutech PLD rectangular W[a]						
4 W	11.5	10	4 × 2			6
6 W	14	12.5	6 × 3			6
8 W	16.5	15	8 × 4			7
10 W	19	17	10 × 4			8
12 W	21	19	12 × 5			9
14 W	24	22	14 × 6			9
16 W	26.5	24.5	16 × 8			10
18 W	28.5	26.5	18 × 10			10
Occlutech PLD rectangular T[b]						
5 T	13	11.5			5 × 3	6
7 T	16	14			7 × 4	7
10 T	19	17			10 × 4	8
12 T	21	19			12 × 5	9
Occlutech PLD square W[a]						
4 W	13	11.5		4		6
5 W	14	12.5		5		6
6 W	16	14		6		6
7 W	17	16		7		7
Occlutech PLD square T[b]						
3 T	11.5	10			3	6
5 T	14	12.5			5	6
7 T	17	16			7	7

[a]*W* waist
[b]*T* twist

Goktekin et al. [29] reported the first use of this device in two patients with mitral and aortic PVLs. Both patients had complete closure. Recently, the same authors have reported a series of 21 consecutive symptomatic patients with moderate or severe paravalvular prosthetic regurgitation who underwent transapical repair with the Occlutech PLD [25]. The patients were followed for 17 ± 5 months. Attempts were made to rectify 41 defects in 21 patients with 100% success. Early post-procedural outcome was uneventful in all cases, with ≥1 grade reduction in regurgitation in all of the patients. There was no mortality during hospital stay. No deaths due to any cause, stroke, or surgery for prosthetic impingement, worsening, or relapse of PVL during follow-up were recorded.

3.5 Selection of the Closure Device

Device choice depends on the shape of the PVLs, the type of prosthetic valve, the access and whether it is planned to use a single or multiple devices. For a small crescent shape PVL, devices such as the AVP III or the Occlutech PLD are used quite frequently. However, for a large crescent shape PVL, a large device (e.g. AmVSDo) can be used, or multiple devices (e.g. AVP III) or sometimes a combination of different devices are needed. In the case of long tunnel-shaped PVLs or "round" PVLs, an AmVSDo or an AVP II could be a good choice, respectively. For a small leak with significant angulation and small neck, an AVP IV occluder is considered. For PVL after TAVI, the AVP IV device is used frequently.

3.6 Paravalvular Mitral Leak Closure with Multiple Devices

In some cases, where one device does not adequately close the PVL, two (or more) devices can be deployed simultaneously or sequentially. To deploy two devices simultaneously, several techniques can be used: (1) Once the PVL has been crossed and the AV loop established, the delivery sheath is advanced through the PVL, and another guide wire is inserted by the delivery sheath. Then, two delivery sheaths are advanced (one on each wire), and the devices are deployed simultaneously (Fig. 3.4a). (2) Deploy a first device without releasing it from the delivery cable, remove the delivery sheath, and advance it again over the "safety" guide wire. After that, a second device is advanced and deployed, and both are released (Fig. 3.4b). (3) Deploy both devices using the same delivery sheath one after the other. In this case, there is risk that the first device can migrate at the time of deploying the second device, and if we do not have a safety wire, it is necessary to cross the PVL again (Fig. 3.4c).

Recently, Smolka G et al. [24] reported the safety and efficacy of PVL closure with simultaneous deployment of multiple AVP III occluders. Forty-nine patients with aortic and mitral PVLs were included. Cumulatively, PVL closure was accomplished in 46 patients (93.9%) with an acute procedural success of 78%. Periprocedural safety endpoints were met in three patients and included non-disabling stroke and two access site-related complications. Significant clinical benefits (reduction of heart failure symptoms and hemolysis) were observed to 30 days and 1 year.

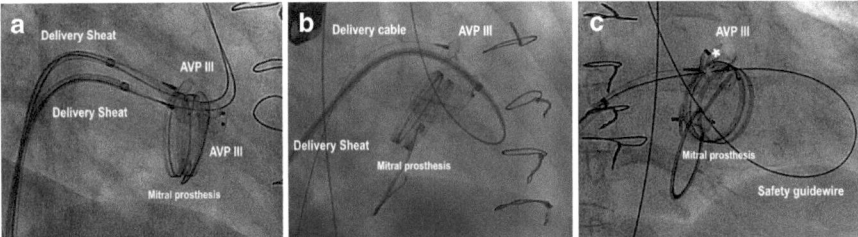

Fig. 3.4 Paravalvular mitral leak closure with multiple devices. (**a**) Two delivery sheaths are advanced (one on each wire), and the devices are deployed simultaneously. (**b**) Deploy a first device without releasing it from the delivery cable, and advance it again over the "safety" guide wire. (**c**) Deploy both devices using the same delivery sheath one after the other (*red* and *white asterisks*)

In our experience, the deployment of multiple "smaller devices" rather than one or two "larger devices" has a better sealing within the PVL and less interference with the prosthesis discs. Also, the adaptation of the devices to the defect is greater when both devices are deployed simultaneously.

3.7 Conclusions and Future Directions

Percutaneous PVL closure is technically a challenging procedure requiring complex catheter techniques and a large interventional armamentarium. At present most devices used for the closure of PVLs are not designed specifically for this purpose, which continues to be a major constraint. For best results, it will be necessary to develop specific devices that are more appropriate to the "complex" anatomy of the PVLs.

References

1. Ionescu A, Fraser AG, Butchart EG. Prevalence and clinical significance of incidental para-prosthetic valvar regurgitation: a prospective study using transoesophageal echocardiography. Heart. 2003;89:1316–21.
2. Genoni M, Franzen D, Vogt P, Seifert B, Jenni R, Kunzli A, Niederhauser U, Turina M. Paravalvular leakage after mitral valve replacement: improved long-term survival with aggressive surgery? Eur J Cardiothorac Surg. 2000;17:14–9.
3. Hammermeister K, Sethi GK, Henderson WG, Grover FL, Oprian C, Rahimtoola SH. Outcomes 15 years after valve replacement with a mechanical versus a bioprosthetic valve: final report of the veterans affairs randomized trial. J Am Coll Cardiol. 2000;36:1152–8.
4. LaPar DJ, Yang Z, Stukenborg GJ, Peeler BB, Kern JA, Kron IL, Ailawadi G. Outcomes of reoperative aortic valve replacement after previous sternotomy. J Thorac Cardiovasc Surg. 2010;139:263–72.
5. Sorajja P, Cabalka AK, Hagler DJ, Rihal CS. Percutaneous repair of paravalvular prosthetic regurgitation: acute and 30-day outcomes in 115 patients. Circ Cardiovasc Interv. 2011;4:314–21.
6. Hein R, Wunderlich N, Robertson G, Wilson N, Sievert H. Catheter closure of paravalvular leak. EuroIntervention. 2006;2:318–25.
7. Cortes M, Garcia E, Garcia-Fernandez MA, Gomez JJ, Perez-David E, Fernandez-Aviles F. Usefulness of transesophageal echocardiography in percutaneous transcatheter repairs of paravalvular mitral regurgitation. Am J Cardiol. 2008;101:382–6.
8. Ruiz CE, Jelnin V, Kronzon I, Dudiy Y, Del Valle-Fernandez R, Einhorn BN, Chiam PT, Martinez C, Eiros R, Roubin G, Cohen HA. Clinical outcomes in patients undergoing percutaneous closure of periprosthetic paravalvular leaks. J Am Coll Cardiol. 2011;58:2210–7.
9. Nietlispach F, Johnson M, Moss RR, Wijesinghe N, Gurvitch R, Tay EL, Thompson C, Webb JG. Transcatheter closure of paravalvular defects using a purpose-specific occluder. JACC Cardiovasc Interv. 2010;3:759–65.
10. Cruz-Gonzalez I, Rama-Merchan JC, Arribas-Jimenez A, Rodriguez-Collado J, Martin-Moreiras J, Cascon-Bueno M, Luengo CM. Paravalvular leak closure with the Amplatzer vascular plug III device: immediate and short-term results. Rev Esp Cardiol (Engl Ed). 2014;67:608–14.

11. Kliger C, Eiros R, Isasti G, Einhorn B, Jelnin V, Cohen H, Kronzon I, Perk G, Fontana GP, Ruiz CE. Review of surgical prosthetic paravalvular leaks: diagnosis and catheter-based closure. Eur Heart J. 2013;34:638–49.
12. Krishnaswamy A, Kapadia SR, Tuzcu EM. Percutaneous paravalvular leak closure- imaging, techniques and outcomes. Circ J. 2013;77:19–27.
13. Kim MS, Casserly IP, Garcia JA, Klein AJ, Salcedo EE, Carroll JD. Percutaneous transcatheter closure of prosthetic mitral paravalvular leaks: are we there yet? JACC Cardiovasc Interv. 2009;2:81–90.
14. Hourihan M, Perry SB, Mandell VS, Keane JF, Rome JJ, Bittl JA, Lock JE. Transcatheter umbrella closure of valvular and paravalvular leaks. J Am Coll Cardiol. 1992;20:1371–7.
15. Lock JE, Cockerham JT, Keane JF, Finley JP, Wakely PE Jr, Fellows KE. Transcatheter umbrella closure of congenital heart defects. Circulation. 1987;75:593–9.
16. Rashkind WJ, Mullins CE, Hellenbrand WE, Tait MA. Nonsurgical closure of patent ductus arteriosus: clinical application of the Rashkind PDA Occluder System. Circulation. 1987;75:583–92.
17. Rashkind WJ. Transcatheter treatment of congenital heart disease. Circulation. 1983;67:711–6.
18. Rome JJ, Keane JF, Perry SB, Spevak PJ, Lock JE. Double-umbrella closure of atrial defects. Initial clinical applications. Circulation. 1990;82:751–8.
19. Lock JE, Rome JJ, Davis R, Van Praagh S, Perry SB, Van Praagh R, Keane JF. Transcatheter closure of atrial septal defects. Experimental studies. Circulation. 1989;79:1091–9.
20. Moore JD, Lashus AG, Prieto LR, Drummond-Webb J, Latson LA. Transcatheter coil occlusion of perivalvular mitral leaks associated with severe hemolysis. Catheter Cardiovasc Interv. 2000;49:64–7.
21. Eisenhauer AC, Piemonte TC, Watson PS. Closure of prosthetic paravalvular mitral regurgitation with the Gianturco-Grifka vascular occlusion device. Catheter Cardiovasc Interv. 2001;54:234–8.
22. Sanchez-Recalde A, Moreno R, Galeote G, Jimenez-Valero S, Calvo L, Sevillano JH, Arroyo-Ucar E, Lopez T, Mesa JM, Lopez-Sendon JL. Immediate and mid-term clinical course after percutaneous closure of paravalvular leakage. Rev Esp Cardiol (Engl Ed). 2014;67:615–23.
23. Shapira Y, Hirsch R, Kornowski R, Hasdai D, Assali A, Vaturi M, Sievert H, Hein R, Battler A, Sagie A. Percutaneous closure of perivalvular leaks with Amplatzer occluders: feasibility, safety, and shortterm results. J Heart Valve Dis. 2007;16:305–13.
24. Smolka G, Pysz P, Jasinski M, Roleder T, Peszek-Przybyla E, Ochala A, Wojakowski W. Multiplug paravalvular leak closure using Amplatzer vascular plugs III: a prospective registry. Catheter Cardiovasc Interv. 2016;87:478–87.
25. Goktekin O, Vatankulu MA, Ozhan H, Ay Y, Ergelen M, Tasal A, Aydin C, Ismail Z, Ates I, Hijazi Z. Early experience of percutaneous paravalvular leak closure using a novel Occlutech occluder. EuroIntervention. 2016;11:1195–200.
26. Sorajja P, Cabalka AK, Hagler DJ, Rihal CS. Long-term follow-up of percutaneous repair of paravalvular prosthetic regurgitation. J Am Coll Cardiol. 2011;58:2218–24.
27. Saia F, Martinez C, Gafoor S, Singh V, Ciuca C, Hofmann I, Marrozzini C, Tan J, Webb J, Sievert H, Marzocchi A, O'Neill WW. Long-term outcomes of percutaneous paravalvular regurgitation closure after transcatheter aortic valve replacement: a multicenter experience. JACC Cardiovasc Interv. 2015;8:681–8.
28. Cruz-Gonzalez I, Rama-Merchan JC, Rodriguez-Collado J, Nieto-Ballestero F, Arribas-Jimenez A, Sanchez PL. Paravalvular leak closure after transcatheter aortic valve implantation simultaneously using Amplatzer vascular plug III and IV devices. Rev Esp Cardiol (Engl Ed). 2015;68:1035–6.
29. Goktekin O, Vatankulu MA, Tasal A, Sonmez O, Basel H, Topuz U, Ergelen M, Hijazi ZM. Transcatheter trans-apical closure of paravalvular mitral and aortic leaks using a new device: first in man experience. Catheter Cardiovasc Interv. 2014;83:308–14.

Chapter 4
Occlutech® Paravalvular Leak Device (PLD)

Eustaquio Maria Onorato, Aleksejus Zorinas, Vilius Janusauskas, Giedrius Davidavicius, Diana Zakarkaite, Rita Kramena, Valdas Bilkis, Kestutis Rucinskas, Robertas Stasys Samalavicius, and Audrius Aidietis

4.1 Background

Since the first reported use of the double-umbrella Rashkind device [1] in 1992, transcatheter paravalvular leak (PVL) closure has been performed extensively by many centers around the world.

A surprising number of different devices including atrial septal defect occluders, duct occluders, muscular ventricular septal defect occluders, and, more recently, vascular plugs [2–11] have been used to close aortic or mitral paravalvular leaks.

E.M. Onorato (✉)
Cardiovascular Department, Humanitas Gavazzeni,
Via Mauro Gavazzeni, 21, 24125 Bergamo, Italy
e-mail: eustaquio.onorato@gmail.com

A. Zorinas • V. Janusauskas • K. Rucinskas
Department of Cardiovascular Medicine, Vilnius University, Vilnius, Lithuania

Centre of Cardiothoracic Surgery, Vilnius University Hospital Santariskiu Klinikos,
Vilnius, Lithuania

G. Davidavicius • D. Zakarkaite • A. Aidietis
Department of Cardiovascular Medicine, Vilnius University, Vilnius, Lithuania

Centre of Cardiology and Angiology, Vilnius University Hospital Santariskiu Klinikos,
Vilnius, Lithuania

R. Kramena
Centre of Cardiology and Angiology, Vilnius University Hospital Santariskiu Klinikos,
Vilnius, Lithuania

V. Bilkis
Department of Cardiovascular Medicine, Vilnius University, Vilnius, Lithuania

R.S. Samalavicius
Department of Intensive Care, Centre of Anaesthesia, Intensive Care, and Pain Management,
Vilnius University, Vilnius, Lithuania

© Springer Nature Singapore Pte Ltd. 2017
G. Smolka et al. (eds.), *Transcatheter Paravalvular Leak Closure*,
DOI 10.1007/978-981-10-5400-6_4

Appearing crescentic shaped in cross sections, PVL entry and exit orifices have diverse morphologies (round, slit-like, oval, or crescentic), and the above devices do not always fit the PVL with subsequent failure of complete closure. This can lead to hemolysis, device embolization, or even coronary occlusions. In addition to the different PVL shapes, paths between the annulus and the sewing ring of the valve have tortuous, irregular, serpiginous courses which can be challenging with regard to wire and catheter crossings and in obtaining an effective seal. Thus, procedural success, defined as a successful deployment of a closure device with stable position without any interference with the prosthetic valve discs/leaflets or acute conversion to surgery, has been impacted by a high incidence of residual shunt and interference of the implanted device with prosthetic leaflets.

A device specifically designed to close PVLs may therefore improve procedural successes and, overall, long-term outcomes. The Occlutech® paravalvular leak device (PLD, manufactured by Occlutech Holding, Switzerland) is a novel device with unique rectangular- and square-shaped designs specifically designed for PVL closure. The Occlutech® PLD was CE marked in 2014 and is the first transcatheter device indicated and approved for aortic and mitral PVL closure.

4.2 Device Description

The Occlutech® PLD obtained CE mark approval on October 7, 2014. The device is made of a nitinol braided wire mesh and is available with square and rectangular disc designs (Figs. 4.1 and 4.2). Rectangular devices are connected by an ellipsoid

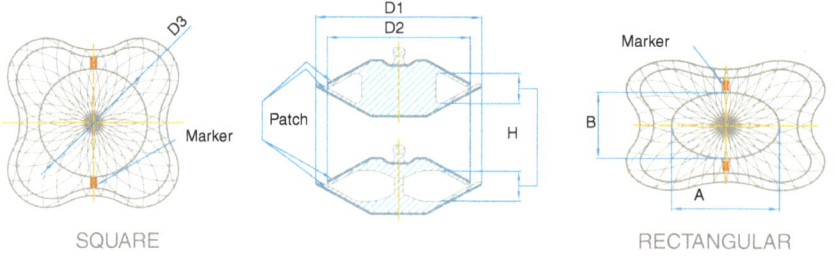

D1 -Length of the distal disc (bigger disc) for PLD	AxB -Length x Width of the waist of rectangular PLD
D2 -Length of the proximal disc (smaller disc) for PLD	H -Height of the waist (3 mm for all sizes)
D3 -Diameter of the waist for square PLD	Min. ID -Recommended minimum inner dimension for delivery sheath

Fig. 4.1 Occlutech® paravalvular leak device (PLD), manufactured by Occlutech Holding, Switzerland: illustrations of the technical characteristics of the square shaped and rectangular shaped in the two different disc connections

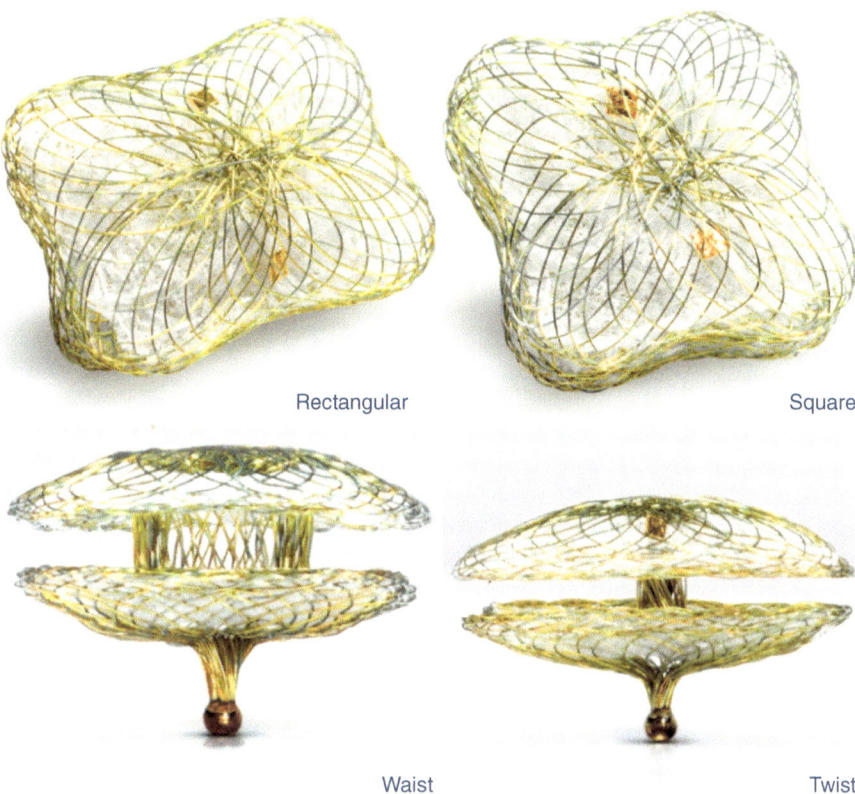

Rectangular   Square

Waist   Twist

Fig. 4.2 Pictures of the two different shapes (*above*) and the two different disc connections (*below*) of the Occlutech® PLD

waist, while square devices have a circular waist. Devices having square discs are intended for closure of circular leaks, while rectangular device designs are intended for crescent-shaped leaks. Two thin polyethylene terephthalate (PET) patches inside of each disc provide for PVL closure immediately after implantation of the device. Two radiopaque gold markers on the distal disc indicate the disc frame location, enhance visibility of the device, and allow for accurate deployment across the defect (Fig. 4.3).

The Occlutech® PLDs are available in sizes ranging from 3 to 7 mm (square designs) that require 6–7 Fr sheaths and from 4 × 2 to 18 × 10 mm (rectangular designs) that require 5–10 Fr sheaths for delivery (Figs. 4.4 and 4.5). The device can be delivered, at the physician's choice, either via transapical or endovascular routes.

Both rectangular and square designs have 35% less surface area as compared to a similar sized, circular design. This reduces the possibility of mechanical interference with a valve and minimizes device overlap in case multiple Occlutech® PLDs are needed to seal a leak.

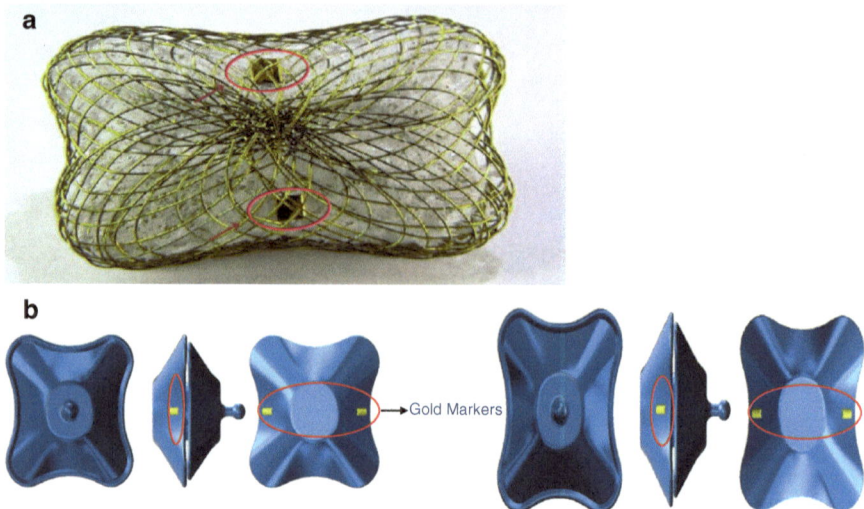

Fig. 4.3 Occlutech® PLD. (**a**) *Red circles* and *arrows* show the two gold radiopaque markers to secure device positioning; (**b**) representative pictures of PLD square (*left*) and of PLD rectangular (*right*): *pictures* from *left* to *right* show the view from the proximal disc, side view, and view from the distal disc, respectively

Occlutech® *PLD RECTANGULAR_W**						
REF NO	**D1 [mm]**	**D2 [mm]**	**AxB [mm]**	**Introducing system ****		**Flex Pusher Item no.**
				ID [mm]	**Size [F]**	
61 PLD 04W	11.5	10	4x2	2.21	6	50FP100L Dark Blue
61 PLD 06W	14	12.5	6x3	2.21	6	50FP100L Dark Blue
61 PLD 08W	16.5	15	8x4	2.54	7	50FP100L Dark Blue
61 PLD 10W	19	17	10x4	2.87	8	50FP100L Dark Blue
61 PLD 12W	21	19	12x5	3.20	9	50FP120L Dark Green
61 PLD 14W	24	22	14x6	3.20	9	50FP120L Dark Green
61 PLD 16W	26.5	24.5	16x8	3.40	10	50FP120L Dark Green
61 PLD 18W	28.5	26.5	18x10	3.40	10	50FP120L Dark Green

Occlutech® *PLD RECTANGULAR_T**						
REF NO	**D1 [mm]**	**D2 [mm]**	**Defect Size [mm]**	**Introducing system size**		**Item no. Flex Pusher**
				Min. ID [mm]	**Size [F]**	
63 PLD 05T	13	11.5	5x3	2.21	6	50FP100 & 50FP100L -dark blue-
63 PLD 07T	16	14	7x4	2.54	7	50FP100 & 50FP100L -dark blue-
63 PLD 10T	19	17	10x4	2.87	8	50FP100 & 50FP100L -dark blue-
63 PLD 12T	21	19	12x5	3.20	9	50FP120 & 50FP120L -dark green-

Occlutech® PLD SQUARE_W						
REF NO	**D1** [mm]	**D2** [mm]	**D3** [mm]	**Introducing system size**		**Item no.** **Flex Pusher**
				Min. ID [mm]	**size[F]**	
60 PLD 04W	13	11.5	4	2.21	6	50FP100 & 50FP100L -dark blue-
60 PLD 05W	14	12.5	5	2.21	6	50FP100 & 50FP100L -dark blue-
60 PLD 06W	16	14	6	2.21	6	50FP100 & 50FP100L -dark blue-
60 PLD 07W	17	16	7	2.54	7	50FP100 & 50FP100L -dark blue-

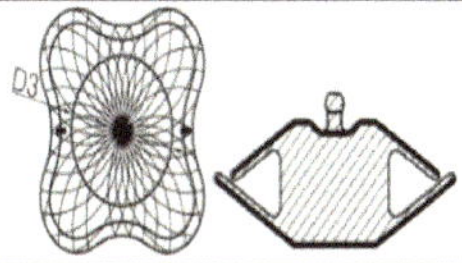

Occlutech® PLD SQUARE_T						
REF NO	**D1** [mm]	**D2** [mm]	**Defect size** [mm]	**Introducing system size**		**Item no.** **Flex Pusher**
				Min. ID [mm]	**size[F]**	
62 PLD 03T	11.5	10	3	2.21	6	50FP100 & 50FP100L -dark blue--
62 PLD 05T	14	12.5	5	2.21	6	50FP100 & 50FP100L -dark blue-
62 PLD 07T	17	16	7	2.54	7	50FP100 & 50FP100L -dark blue-

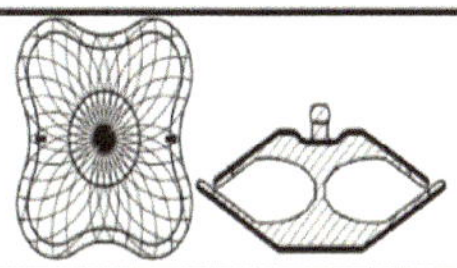

Fig. 4.5 Occlutech® **square** PLD: recommended delivery systems and devices sizes. W and T represent the types of connections between the discs. W stands for waist (D3 or $A \times B$); T stands for twist (connection diameter is negligible) * and ** = Availability subject to regulatory approval

Moreover, due to the waist designs, the Occlutech® PLD has no radial strength, but it has an intrinsic clamping force that keeps the prosthetic valve and tissue in close proximity to each other after PVL closure. In contrast, vascular plugs of Amplatzer family have high radial strength (large waists) and lack the clamping force (e.g., Amplatzer Vascular Plug III).

The Occlutech® PLD wire braiding ends in a welded ball on the proximal side of the device. This ball serves as adapter for the pusher cable (Flex Pusher, manufactured by Occlutech Holding, Switzerland, Fig. 4.6a, b). To connect an

Fig. 4.4 Occlutech® **rectangular** PLD: recommended delivery systems and devices sizes. W and T represent the types of connections between the discs. W stands for waist (D3 or $A \times B$); T stands for twist (connection diameter is negligible) * and ** = Availability subject to regulatory approval

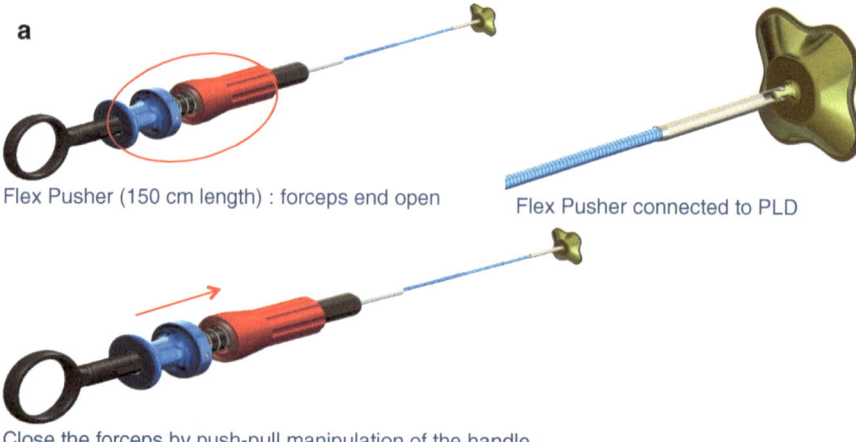

a Flex Pusher (150 cm length) : forceps end open

Flex Pusher connected to PLD

Close the forceps by push-pull manipulation of the handle

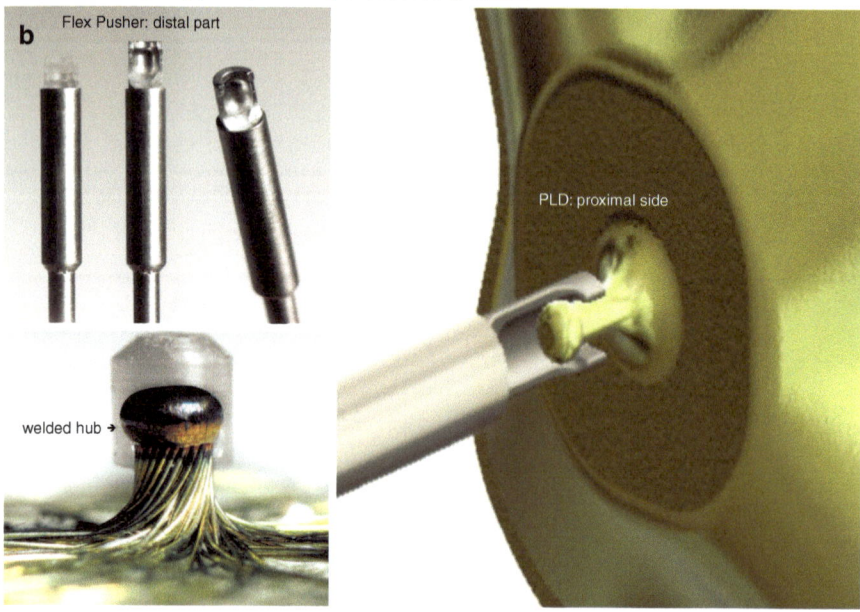

b Flex Pusher: distal part

welded hub →

PLD: proximal side

Fig. 4.6 (**a**) The Flex Pusher and PLD: the handle of the cable untightened (*left upper*); Flex Pusher connected to PLD (*right upper*); to prevent premature release of the device, the handle of the cable is tightened acting as a security mechanism (*below*). (**b**) On the proximal side of the PLD, the wire braiding ends in a welded hub which connect to the distal part of the Flex Pusher in a socket sleeve, somewhat similar to a bioptome. (**c**) The Flex Pusher connected to the PLD and locked. (**d**) The handle of the cable is untightened in order to release the device by pushing the handle, once the PLD is in good position

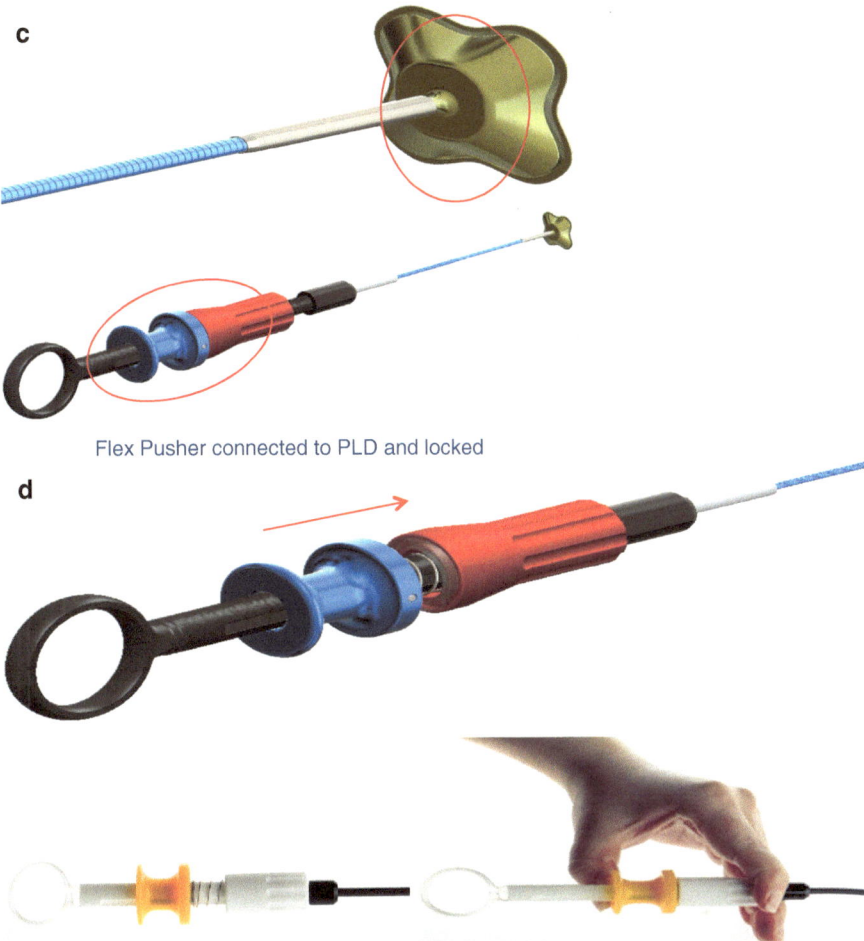

c

Flex Pusher connected to PLD and locked

d

Loosen the locking mechanism and push / pull function of the handle in order to release PLD

Fig.4.6 (continued)

Occlutech® PLD to the Flex Pusher, the handle of the pusher is pulled back to open the jaws located at the distal end of the wire. Release of the handle causes the jaw to close around the ball adapter thus attaching the pusher wire to the device. Once attached, the connection is secured by means of actuating a screw (locking mechanism) on the handle of the pusher to prevent accidental or premature release of the device (Fig. 4.6c). After the Occlutech® PLD has been positioned optimally in the PVL area, the device can be disconnected from its pusher cable by loosening the locking mechanism and releasing the handle (Fig. 4.6d).

4.3   Implantation Procedure

Transcatheter PVL closure device delivery techniques vary significantly among physicians and/or centers. Notwithstanding, the procedure is performed in a hybrid operating room with the patient under general anesthesia and using fluoroscopic and transesophageal echocardiographic (TEE) guidance (see Sect. 4.4).

On the day of the procedure, standard endocarditis prophylaxis (e.g., second- to fourth-generation cephalosporin) is administered. Patients are anticoagulated with 60–100 IU of unfractionated heparin/kg to achieve an activated clotting time (ACT) of ≥ 250 s.

4.3.1   Mitral Paravalvular Leaks

General considerations:

1. Mitral PVL repair is technically more demanding when compared to aortic PVL, and close cooperation between the imaging team and interventionalists is of paramount importance. Due to the extensive manipulation in the left atrium, generous anticoagulation should be administered (e.g., ACT ≥ 300 s).
2. A careful *preprocedural analysis* of leak size, number, and location using 2D/3D TEE and 4D computed tomography angiography (4D-CTA) should be performed. When selecting the size of the device, it is highly recommended not to oversize the occluder in order to avoid excessive distortion of the device and interference with the neighboring structures.
3. For laterally located leaks (9–11 o'clock, Figs. 4.7 and 4.8), an *anterograde approach* should be taken. Transseptal puncture is a key step in this approach. After positioning of the delivery sheath in the right femoral vein, a transseptal puncture is performed by maneuvering a 5 Fr multipurpose catheter via a steerable/deflectable sheath. Next, the mitral paravalvular leak is crossed from the left atrium into the left ventricle. The Occlutech® PLD can now be advanced using a delivery sheath, and the leak can be closed.
4. For anteriorly located leaks (12–1 o'clock, Fig. 4.8 and 4.9a), a *retrograde approach* can be useful. A catheter is inserted into the femoral artery and guided through the left ventricle into the left atrium using a Judkins Left or Right catheter. A hydrophilic wire is then used to trans-navigate the leak and to cross into to the left atrium. Frequently, this wire needs to be snared and exteriorized from the femoral vein; thus, an arteriovenous loop to advance the sheath from the femoral vein (anterograde) should be established. The Occlutech® PLD can now be advanced using a delivery sheath, and the leak can be closed.
5. The *transapical route* (Fig. 4.9b) is our preferred approach, particularly for anteromedially, posteromedially, and posterolaterally located leaks (2–8 o'clock, Fig. 4.7). This procedure requires a limited thoracotomy that is performed by a cardiac surgeon. Once the left ventricular apex has been identified, the left ventricle is punctured

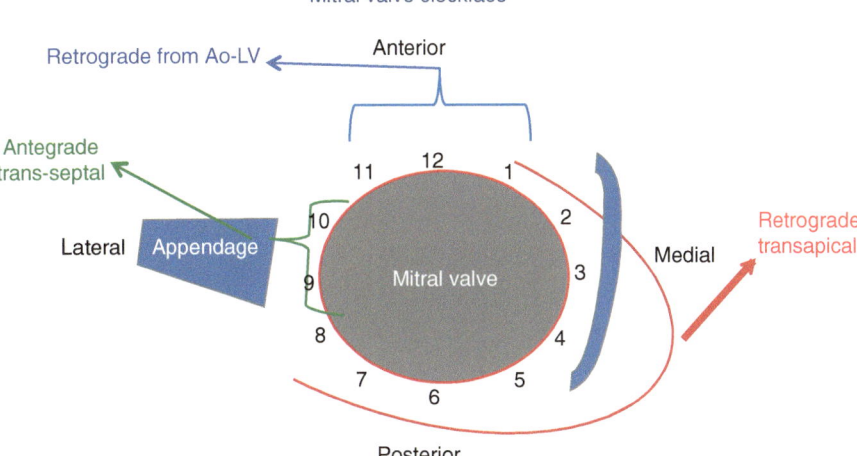

Fig. 4.7 Mitral valve clockface. Recommended approaches for transcatheter PVL closure based on the location of the leaks

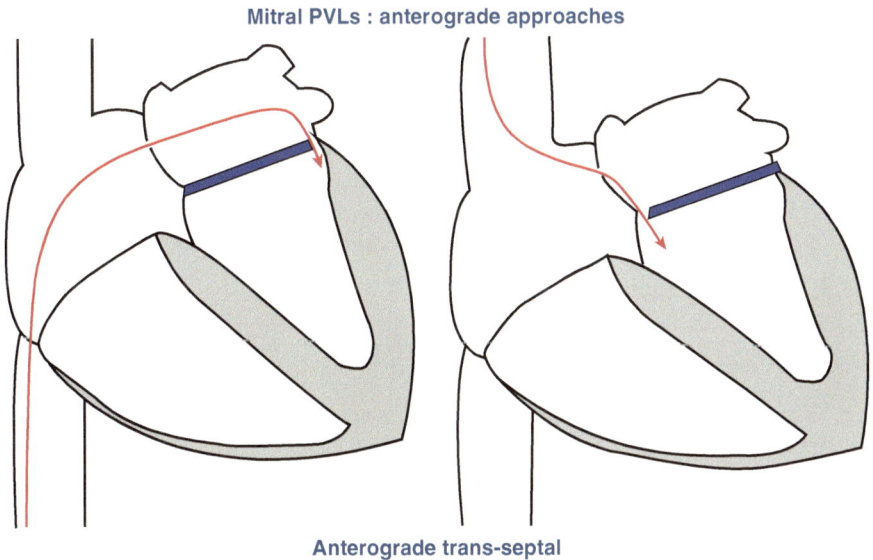

Fig. 4.8 Antegrade approaches for closing prosthetic mitral PVLs. Advantages and disadvantages

Mitral PVLs : retrograde approaches

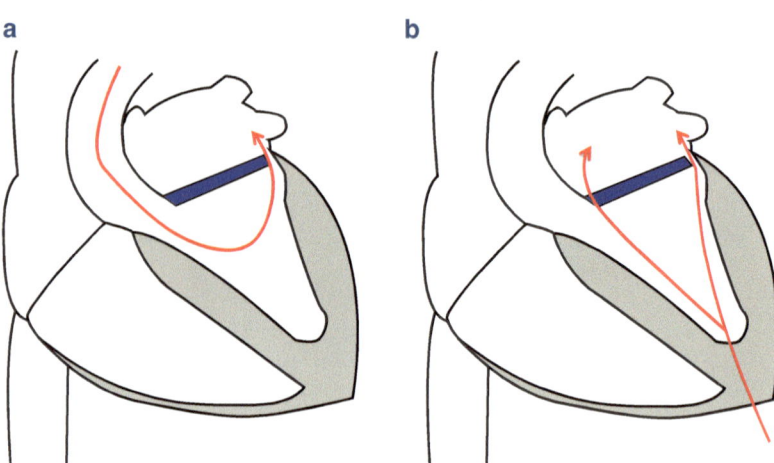

a   **b**

Retrograde from Aorta-Left Ventricle   **Trans-apical**

Crossing *on the same direction* of the regurgitant flow through the leak, better wire *pushability*,
transapical approach more invasive

Fig. 4.9 Retrograde approaches for closing prosthetic mitral PVLs. (**a**) Retrograde from aorta-left ventricle; (**b**) retrograde transapical. Advantages and disadvantages

in a position parallel to that of the leak. A short sheath is inserted into the left ventricle, the leak is crossed, and the sheath is placed into the left atrium. The Occlutech® PLD can now be advanced using a delivery sheath, and the leak can be closed.

4.3.2 Aortic Paravalvular Leaks

General considerations:

1. Generally, percutaneous aortic PVL repair is not technically difficult, and it should be considered as the first therapeutic option in these patients as opposed to surgery.
2. Aortic PVLs are most often located near the non-coronary sinus, and percutaneous repair of aortic PVLs is feasible in most patients (Fig. 4.10).
3. Two-dimensional color Doppler and real-time 3D TEE are necessary. Angiography of the ascending aorta in different planes is used to define the location of the aortic leak and to guide the procedure and validate the outcomes.
4. A *retrograde approach* (via the femoral artery) is the most common route of intervention. In some cases, a *retrograde transapical approach* may also be used particularly in cases of calcified, tortuous, and elongated aortic arch and thoraco-abdominal aortic aneurysm. In this abovementioned setting of patients, even a retrograde transaortic approach (via the subclavian artery) represents an alternate route of intervention. Brachial access can be also used and may become a more established procedure used with the Occlutech® PLD in the near future (Fig. 4.11).

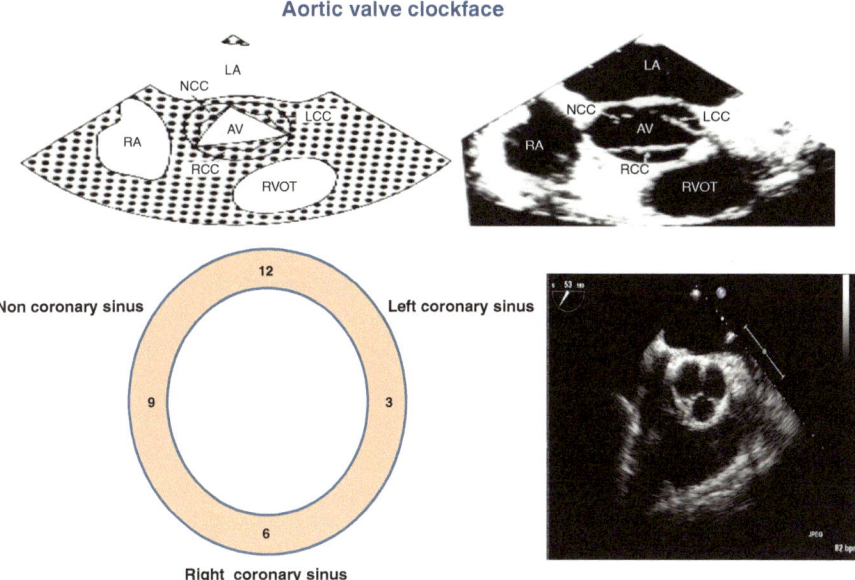

Fig. 4.10 Aortic valve clockface with corresponding TEE imaging and a schematic pattern. Aortic PVLs are most often located near the non-coronary sinus

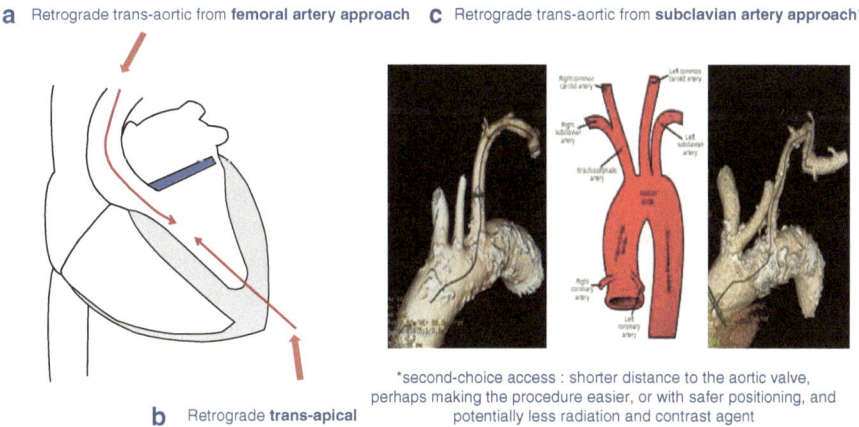

Fig. 4.11 Retrograde approaches for transcatheter closure of aortic PVLs. (**a**) Retrograde trans-aortic from femoral artery; (**b**) retrograde transapical; (**c**) retrograde trans-aortic from subclavian artery. Subclavian artery approach could be an alternative second-choice access in cases of severely calcified, tortuous, and elongated aortic arch and thoraco-abdominal aortic aneurysm

5. Access through the leak can be accomplished by first using a multipurpose catheter and a hydrophilic wire. Once the leak is crossed, the hydrophilic wire is exchanged for a 0.035-in. stiff wire with a soft tip. This latter wire is introduced and placed to rest in either the left ventricle (retrograde approach) or in the ascending aorta (transapical approach). The Occlutech® PLD can now be advanced using a delivery sheath, and the leak can be closed.

4.4 Pre-, Intra-, and Postprocedural Imaging (See Cases Illustrations)

Although echocardiography is the technique of choice to identify and quantify PVL, additional preprocedural imaging modalities such as ECG-gated computed tomography with three- or four-dimensional (3D/4D CT) reconstruction and magnetic resonance imaging (MRI) scan can be useful providing further details regarding leak's location, number, size, shape, and spatial orientation (planning for transapical access), width and length of the channel, and the assessment of regurgitant volumes.

Performing catheter-based procedures requires the use of numerous imaging modalities and techniques. Thus, access to adequate imaging tools is the cornerstone for making a proper diagnosis, for intraprocedural monitoring, and for assessing and follow-up of postprocedural results.

Accurate, imaging-based assessment of PVL anatomy is a prerequisite, and the use of fluoroscopic imaging is imperative. Orthogonal fluoroscopy views of multiple planes are needed to assure accurate wire placement and PVL closure. Bioprosthetic or mechanical prosthetic valves may be used as reference points during the entire procedure.

Having a comprehensive view of the PVL is crucial for adequate device selection and to determine the best route for implantation. 2D/3D TEE imaging can be used to localize the leak and to assess the number, size, and shape of leaks. Real-time 3D TEE provides more accurate morphological information compared to 2D TEE.

While color Doppler-based imaging modalities to detect and grade regurgitant jet volume are most often used to diagnose and assess the severity of PVLs, TEE is recommended as the most sensitive method. 3D TEE imaging used alone, or used together with 3D color Doppler imaging, is highly accurate to locate PVLs.

In practice and for the ease and clarity of communication among specialists, it is recommended to record the location of a PVL in clockwise fashion from a surgeon's perspective of the valve (Figs. 4.7 and 4.10).

Selecting the right size and shape of an Occlutech® PLD depends on the anatomy of the leak. Images acquired from 2D, 3D, color Doppler, and TEE imaging modalities should be combined to detail the cross-sectional configuration of PVLs (oval, round, or crescent shaped) as well as the shape and length of the leak (flat or tunnel-like).

To precisely measure PVL dimensions, cropped 3D echocardiography datasets to visualize the regurgitant jet volume at the level of the defect or multiplane reconstructions of regurgitant jet volumes followed by vena contracta measurements are utilized.

Traditionally, fluoroscopy imaging has been used to monitor and control the delivery of wires, catheters, and occluders to a desired anatomical site of the heart. More recently, real-time 3D TEE imaging has gained more widespread use due to its obvious benefits. This imaging technique allows interventionalists to precisely guide and monitor the movement of intracardiac devices, as well as the delivery and positioning of occluders to a specific anatomical surrounding.

The newly developed approach entailing the fusion of fluoroscopy and real-time 3D TEE helps in navigating intracardiac tools and crossing defects in PVL closure procedures. This technique is extremely useful in cases when prosthetic valves are invisible under fluoroscopy.

All TEE imaging modalities, as well as fluoroscopy with or without contrast agent, can be utilized to evaluate the position of the occluder, its relation to the prosthesis, and any residual paravalvular leak.

4.5 Clinical Experience

Unlike other devices used off-label for PVL closure, the Occlutech® PLD is specifically indicated for patients with PVL-associated hemolysis, recurrent blood transfusions, or hemodynamically significant heart failure and who are deemed at high risk for surgical intervention after consultation with surgical physicians or as an alternative to surgery with less operational time and recovery period.

Patients with high-risk features for recurrent paravalvular leak, such as severe annular calcification, are also good candidates.

Each PVL is unique in shape, geometry, size, and proximity to the valve prosthesis. As discussed, the shape of PVLs is often crescentic and generally complex. Oblong devices, such as the Occlutech® PLD, may fit PVL defects more accurately.

Rectangular-shaped devices are especially useful for edge repair in crescentic leaks, whereas square-shaped devices seal the center of the regurgitant orifice. In cases with large crescent-shaped defects requiring multiple devices, implantation of rectangular devices to the edges increases the success rate and lowers residual regurgitation without interfering with the valve.

The first in man experience using the Occlutech® PLD was published in 2014 by Goktekin et al. [12]. The two cases performed highlighted the versatility of this new occluder. In the aortic case, a square-shaped device with a round waist was needed, and in the mitral case, a rectangular-shaped device was important to cover the crescent-shaped defect, and in both complete closure was achieved.

In a recent paper by Calvert et al., the use of this kind of devices was associated with less residual leaks as well as with a greater reduction in NYHA class at follow-up [8]. Similarly, Ercan et al. reported high procedural and clinical success rates using the Occlutech® PLD [13].

Again, Goktekin et al. [14] reported the midterm outcomes of percutaneous leak closure with Occlutech® PLD in 21 consecutive symptomatic patients with moderate or severe paravalvular prosthetic regurgitation. The patients were followed for

17 ± 5 months. Attempts were made to treat 41 defects in 21 patients with 100% success. Mean procedural time was 76 ± 40 min and fluoroscopy time was 44 ± 37 min. Early postprocedural outcome was uneventful in all cases, with ≥ 1 grade reduction in regurgitation in all of the patients. There was no mortality during hospital stay. Postimplantation 90-day follow-up data were obtained for 19 patients, and 12-month data were obtained for 12 patients. No deaths due to any cause, stroke, or surgery for prosthetic impingement, worsening, or relapse of paravalvular leak during follow-up were recorded.

In a prospective two-center study [15] between April 2012 and January 2015, 52 patients who needed surgical reintervention due to a hemodynamically significant prosthetic paravalvular leak were studied and divided in two groups. In Group I, 32 patients underwent PVL closure with the currently available devices that are being utilized off-label, while in Group II 20 patients were treated with the new Occlutech® PLD. The apical approach was the most commonly used intervention route used for Group II. The procedural success rate was 100% (29 of 29 leaks) in Group II, while the rate was 92% (39 of 42 leaks) in Group I. Valve interference and defect enlargement causing significant residual leak had an adverse impact on the 6-month outcomes in Group I, while Group II patients were free of such undesirable outcomes, and, finally, a significant improvement in both 6-min walk test (6MWT) and NYHA class was achieved.

Furthermore, in 2016 Smolka et al. [16] published initial, short-term results from 30 patients, mean age 63 years (range 59–70), with 34 PVLs (16 mitral and 18 aortic) enrolled in a prospective registry to assess the safety and efficacy of PVL closure with the Occlutech® PLD. Twenty-three patients (36.5%) were in NYHA class II/IV, and four (13.2%) had transfusion-depending hemolytic anemia. The mitral location of the PVL was associated with longer procedural time, higher dose of radiation, and lower procedural success rate, particularly if the transseptal approach was performed. Total device success rate was 94.3% (88.2% for mitral, 100% for aortic), and procedural success rate without in-hospital complications was 94.1% (93.8% for mitral, 100% for aortic). There was one case of device failure with exacerbation of hemolytic anemia. No major adverse cardiac and cerebrovascular events occurred during the hospital stay. At 30-day follow-up, no additional events were noted, and none of the patients required transfusion, while the NYHA class was I in 14 patients (46.6%), II in 13 patients (43.3%), and III in 3 patients (10%). The authors concluded that a meticulous preselection of patients based on imaging of PVL anatomy is a prerequisite, and device size should match the PVL cross-sectional area without any oversizing.

In 2015, we have initiated a prospective, international, multicenter follow-up study to assess the safety and efficacy of percutaneous closure of mitral and aortic PVLs by the Occlutech® PLD. As of January 2017, 50 patients, average age 66.5 years, range 26–88, 31 (64.6%) males, with severe symptomatic (heart failure, hemolytic anemia, or both) paravalvular regurgitation underwent transcatheter PVL closure with Occlutech® PLD in 17 European centers (see Appendix). There were 40 mitral (80%) and 10 aortic (20%) PVLs and 62% of the leaks were crescent-shaped. Implantation of the device was successfully accomplished in 48 patients (96%). Preliminary results from 28 (56%) patients at midterm follow-up (12 months) showed a reduction in paravalvular regurgitation by one grade or more (echocardiography) and/or a reduction in the number of hemolysis-related transfusions in more than 60% of the patients treated. No late device embolizations or other serious adverse events occurred thus far. While the total number of patients is still small and follow-up incomplete, these results are encouraging.

In the setting of the abovementioned international, multicenter follow-up study, the clinical experience particularly at Vilnius University Hospital Santariskiu Klinikos, in Vilnius, Lithuania, confirmed undoubtedly that transapical approach has proven practical and feasible and has resulted in high rates of mitral PVL closures. Indeed, this approach allows access to leaks at all anatomic locations of mitral valve prostheses [17]. In addition, the fusion of fluoroscopy and real-time 3D TEE helped in navigating intracardiac tools and crossing defects in PVL closure procedures (see Cases Illustrations). This technique turned out to be extremely useful in cases when prosthetic valves are invisible under fluoroscopy.

4.6   Summary

Transcatheter PVL closure is an effective but a technically demanding procedure with a steep learning curve. Interventionalists must master complex cardiac catheterization techniques involving a large armamentarium of transcatheter devices, gain experience with multiple imaging modalities, and develop the skills to visualize the 3D relationships of intracardiac structures. Indeed, collaborative efforts among skilled interventionalists, surgeons, and an experienced imaging team are imperative to perform successful PVL closures.

The Occlutech® PLD has demonstrated remarkably high procedural success rates, and preliminary outcome results from the literature and also from the ongoing prospective, international, multicenter follow-up study are encouraging. This is most likely due to the specific device design that, with two shapes (square and rectangular) and two different disc connections (waist and twist), may be more adaptable to and/or conform better to different PVL shapes, thereby providing a greater range of possibilities for full coverage of the leaks and a glimmer of hope after a long course of marginal success with the previous off-label vascular plugs.

Novel transcatheter approaches to close complex PVLs are also improving procedural success and reduce complication rates. As shown, integration of multimodal imaging techniques (fusion imaging modalities) in the catheter lab together with a mini-thoracotomy apical approach for mitral PVLs [17–19] provides the potential to further advance and de-risk this otherwise challenging transcatheter procedure.

Although transcatheter closure with Occlutech® PLD is a viable therapeutic alternative to surgical PVL repair, even for highest-risk symptomatic PVL patients, long-term mortality rates, however, remain high, thus confirming the high-risk profile of these patients who, in addition to PVLs, suffer from multiple and serious comorbidities (previous cardiac surgeries, COPD, chronic renal failure, old age, and frailty).

Clinical and echocardiographic long-term follow-up data and larger patient series will be useful to improve even more the technical success of the procedure, to guide more general adoption of this new purpose-specific technology in order to provide sufficient data for scientific assessment of clinical success.

Acknowledgments We are indebted to the staff of the catheter lab at Vilnius University, Lithuania, for their help during the procedures. We are extremely grateful to Lina Puodziukaite and Rokas Simakauskas for their efforts in data collection (both are medical students in Vilnius University). The authors also thank the engineering and marketing staff at Occlutech for illustrations, for technical descriptions of the device, and for their continuing logistic support.

Conflict of Interest Statement Dr. Eustaquio Maria Onorato is a Consultant for Occlutech, manufacturer of the device, and Co-Principal Investigator of the international, multicenter follow-up study to monitor the efficacy and safety of the Occlutech® paravalvular leak device (PLD) in patients with mitral or aortic paravalvular leaks (see Appendix).

The remaining authors have no conflicts of interest to declare.

Cases Illustrations

1. Preprocedural (*red area*) and postprocedural (*green area*) color Doppler TEE images for three cases of PVL closure. Case 1, Case 2, and Case 3 show the single mitral, double mitral, and aortic PVL closure accordingly. Postprocedural images show only trace residual regurgitant jets (*arrows*).

   TEE transesophageal echocardiography, *LA* left atrium, *LV* left ventricle, *RA* right atrium, *RV* right ventricle, *Ao* aorta

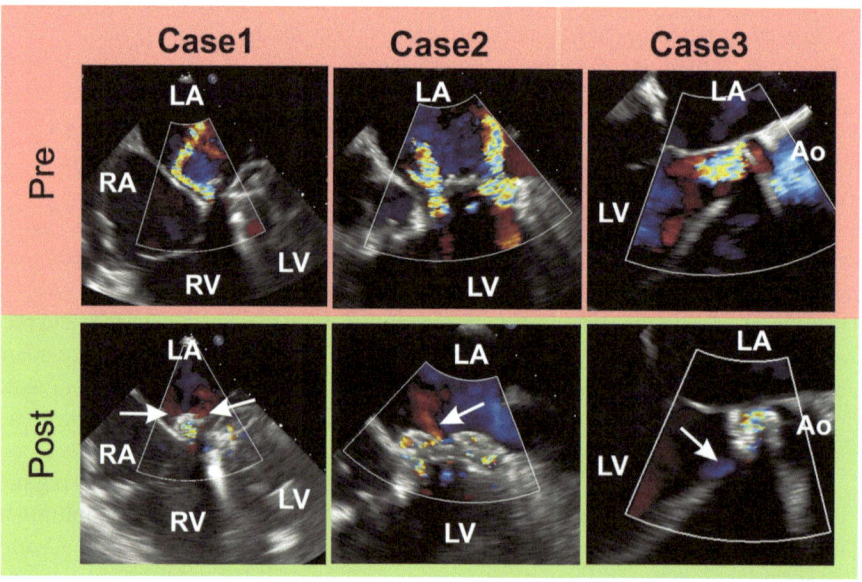

2. The same three cases are presented by TEE images during the procedure. Preprocedural (*red area*) 3D images and 3D color Doppler images cropped at level of the vena contracta clearly identified the single mitral paraprosthetic defect at 2 o'clock position in Case 1, the two mitral PVLs at 10 and 2 o'clock position in Case 2, and the aortic PVL at the noncoronary cusp projection in Case 3 (*arrows*). The first intraprocedural step—the wire crossing the PVL hole (*arrows*)—is nicely seen on 3D images in all cases (*yellow area*).

   As the results of the following case-specific intraprocedural manipulations, all PVLs were closed (*green area*) with only trace residual regurgitant jets (*arrows*). The occluders are marked by *stars*, and the final orientation of the occluders is clearly seen. The occluder position is strongly parallel to the prosthesis edge in Case 1. In Case 2 the right one occluder was fixed perpendicularly because this orientation accomplished the best result. In Case 3 the occluder position is oblique.

TEE transesophageal echocardiography, *P* valve prosthesis, *Ao* aorta

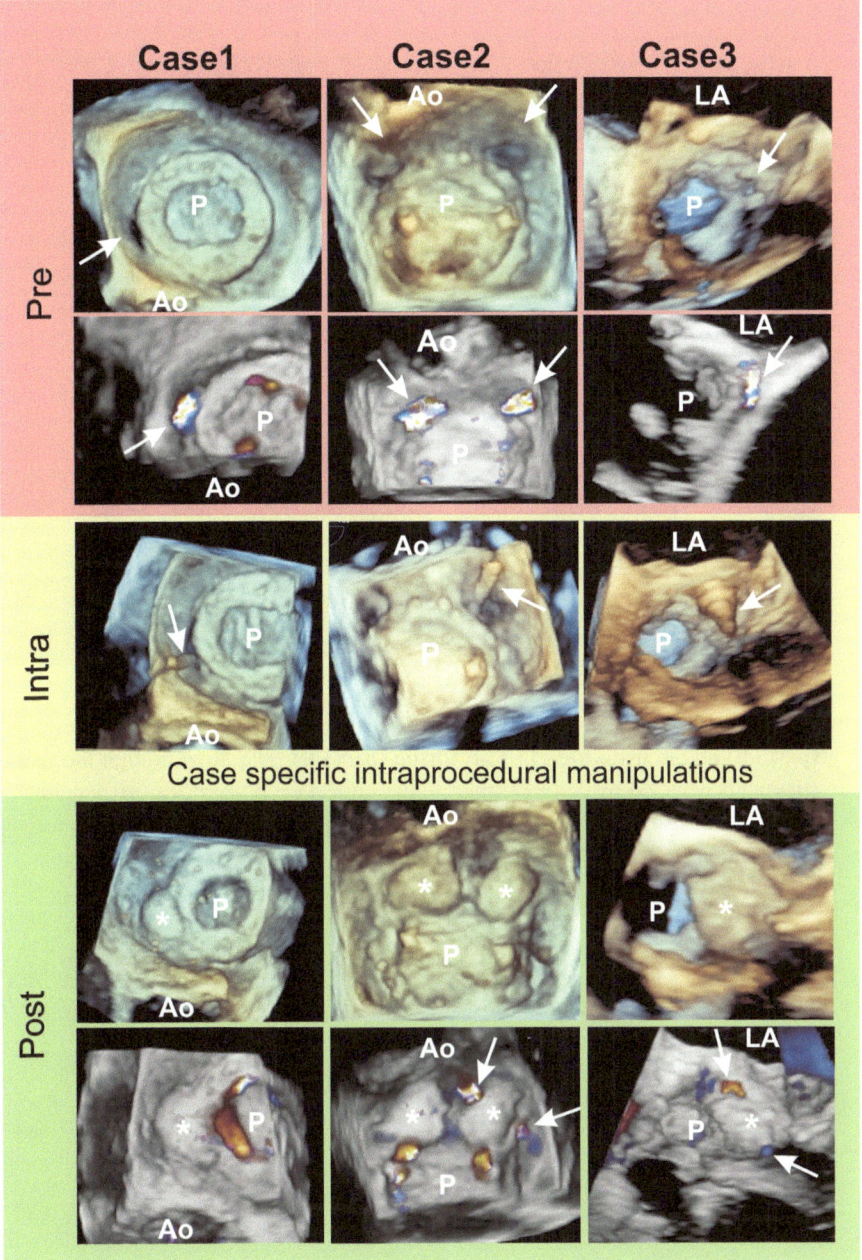

3. The 2D and color Doppler TEE images show the principles of the PVL measurements (*arrows*) in the case of flat (panel **a**) and tunnel (panel **b**) shape of the hole. The precise measurements (*arrows*) of the PVL performed by the cropping of regurgitant jet volume on 3D color Doppler TEE image (panel **b**) or using the multiplane reconstruction of same regurgitant jet volume at the level of the hole (panel **b**).

   TEE transesophageal echocardiography, *P* valve prosthesis, *LA* left atrium, *LV* left ventricle

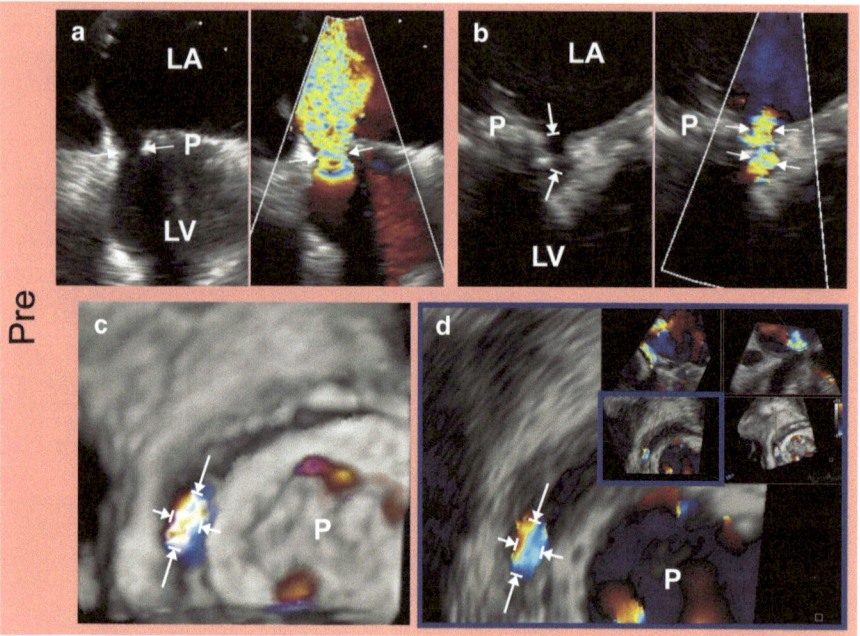

4. The "U"-shaped tunnel-like aortic PVL (*arrows*) is seen on computed tomography (panel **a**) and transgastric 2D TEE image (panel **b**). The flow through the tunnel (*arrow*) is detected by color Doppler in the same TEE probe position (panel **c**).

   TEE transesophageal echocardiography, *P* valve prosthesis, *LV* left ventricle, *RV* right ventricle, *Ao* aorta

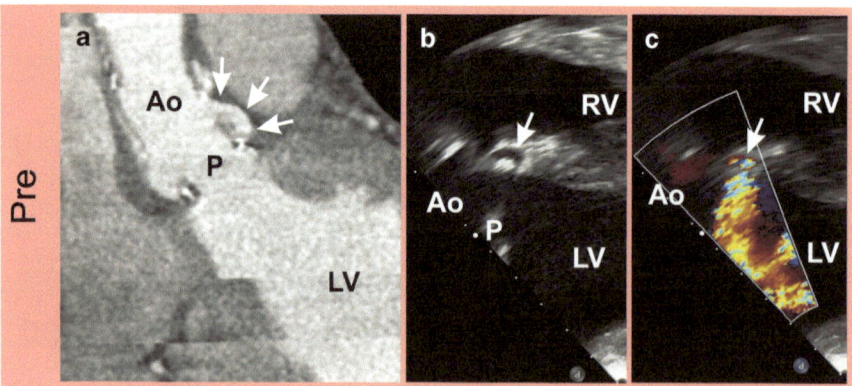

5. The case of transapical transcatheter closure of complex mitral PVL illustrating how extremely helpful is the real-time 3D TEE during the procedure. The case depicted by pre-, intra-, and postprocedural 3D and 3D color Doppler TEE images (*red*, *yellow*, and *green areas*) and by cardiac fluoroscopy images (*blue area*). The two quite close located leaks (*arrows*) and two regurgitant jets were detected before the procedure (panel **a** and **b**). The first wire crossed the right leak (panel **c**). The second wire (*arrows*) fell in to the same leak and finally was placed into the left leak (panel **d** and **e**). The left leak was closed by the first occluder, a RW 8 × 4 mm (panel **f** and **m**) with a significant residual jet (*arrow* on the panel **g**). The right leak was completely closed by the second occluder, a SW 5 mm (panel **h** and **n**). A residual jet from the left leak was still observed (panel **i**). The third wire was passed surrounding the left leak (panel **j** and **o**), and the third occluder, a ST 5 mm, was implanted (panel **k** and **r**). Only two trace residual jets (*arrows*) were present after the procedure (panel **l**).

TEE transesophageal echocardiography, *P* valve prosthesis, *asterisk* occluder, *RW* rectangular waist, *SW* square waist, *ST* square twist

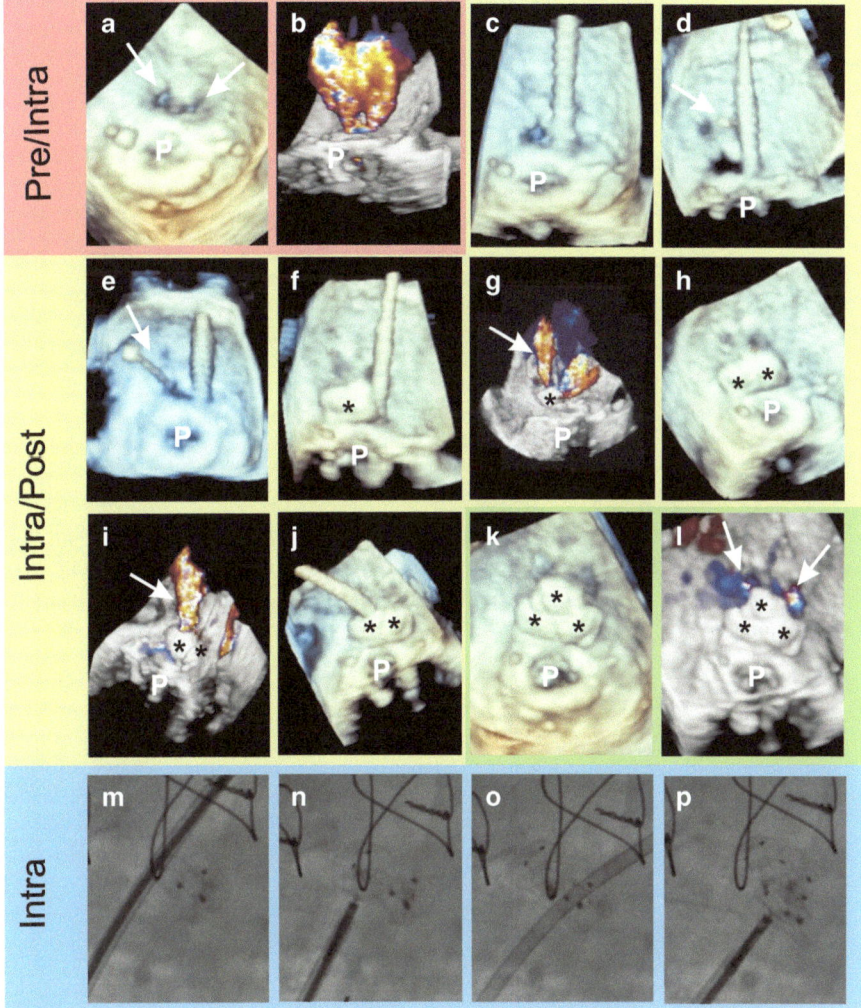

6. The fusion of cardiac fluoroscopy and different TEE modalities.

(**a**)—The multiplane TEE image (on *top*) with *red point* dropped on the place of PVL is fused in the space with fluoroscopic image (on *bottom*). The *green oval* depicts the mitral prosthesis position. The wire is directed to the *red point* on the image.

(**b**)—The multiplane color Doppler image (on *top*) fused with fluoroscopy (on *bottom*) helps to visualize the PVL position signed by *red point*.

(**c**)—The fusion image of 3D TEE image shows the right position of all three PVLs. The wire is crossing the one of them signed as *green point*.

TEE transesophageal echocardiography, *P* valve prosthesis

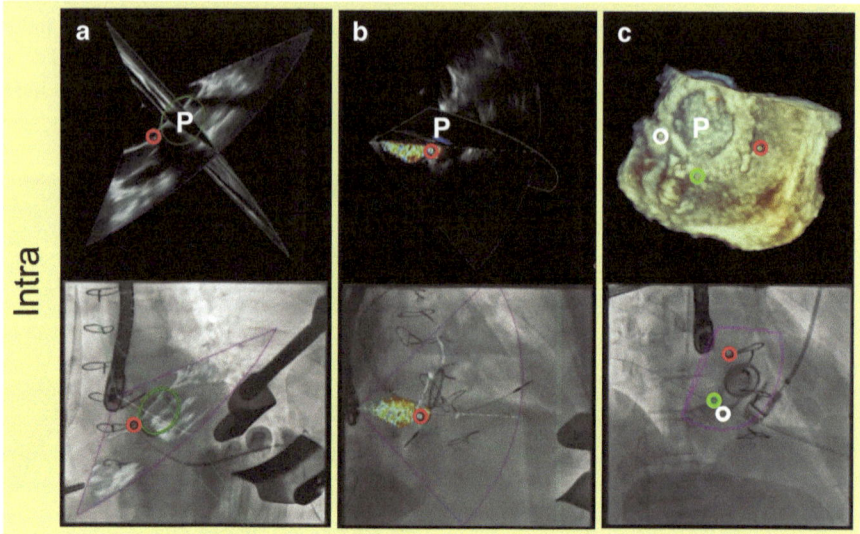

Appendix

The countries, institutions, and investigators participating in the international, multicenter follow-up study to monitor the efficacy and safety of the Occlutech® paravalvular leak device (PLD) in patients with mitral or aortic paravalvular leaks are listed here.

Coordinating Principal Investigators

Dr Eustaquio Maria Onorato, Cardiovascular Department, Humanitas Gavazzeni, Bergamo, Italy, and Prof Shakeel Ahmed Qureshi, Evelina Children's Hospital, London, UK.

Italy

Humanitas Gavazzeni, Bergamo (Dr EM Onorato, Dr A Pitì, Dr F Santoro, Dr M Pennesi)

Centro Cardiologico Monzino, Università degli Studi di Milano (Prof. AL Bartorelli, Prof. F Alamanni, Dr G Tamborini, Dr M Muratori)

Clinica San Gaudenzio, Novara (Dr G Martinelli, Dr G. Cerin, Dr G Carosio, Dr M Diena)

Clinica San Michele, Maddaloni (Dr A De Bellis, Dr P Landino)

Clinica Montevergine, Mercogliano (Av) (Dr T Tesorio, Dr M Agrusta, Dr E Mango)

Città di Alessandria, Policlinico di Monza (Dr M Fabbrocini, Dr P Cioffi)

Azienda Ospedaliera SS. Antonio e Biagio e Cesare Arrigo, Alessandria (Dr M Reale, Dr M Vercellino, Dr AM Costante, Dr G Pistis, Dr D Mercogliano)

Dipartimento di Malattie Cardiovascolari, Campobasso (Dr CM De Filippo, Dr P Spatuzza, Dr E Caradonna)

USVD Emodinamica, Spedali Civili di Brescia (Dr F. Ettori, Dr S. Curello)

Lithuania

Santariskiu Klinikos, Vilnius (Dr A Aidietis, Dr A Zorinas, Dr Vilius Janusauskas, Dr Kestutis Rucinskas, Dr D Zakarkaite, Dr R Kramena, Dr V Bilkis)

France

Centre Hospitalier Universitaire, "Charles Nicole," Rouen (Prof P-Y Litzer, Prof H Eltchaninoff, Dr M Godin, Dr F Bauer, Prof F Doguet)

Centre Hospitalier Universitaire, Hôpital Arnaud de Villeneuve, Montpellier (Prof B Albat, Dr T Grandet, Dr JC Macia, Dr F Cransac)

Centre Hospitalier Régional Universitaire, Lille (Prof F Godart, Prof F Juthier)

Cyprus

American Heart Institute, Nicosia (Dr C Christou, Dr S Constantinides, Dr M Neofytou)

Hungary

National Heart Center, Budapest (Prof A Szatmari, Dr G Fontos)

Romania

Centru Cardiovascular Monza, Bucharest (Prof S Balanescu, Dr A Linte)

UK

Castle Hill Hospital, Cottingham (Dr K Aznaouridis, Dr K Masoura, Dr D Ngaage)

References

1. Hourihan M, Perry SB, Mandell VS, Keane JF, Rome JJ, Bittl JA, et al. Transcatheter umbrella closure of valvular and paravalvular leaks. J Am Coll Cardiol. 1992;20:1371–7.
2. Kim MS, Casserly IP, Garcia JA, Klein AJ, Salcedo EE, Carroll JD. Percutaneous transcatheter closure of prosthetic mitral paravalvular leaks: are we there yet ? JACC Cardiovasc Interv. 2009;2:81–90.
3. Ruiz CE, Jelnin V, Kronzon I, Dudiy Y, Del ValleFernandez R, Einhorn BN, et al. Clinical outcomes in patients undergoing percutaneous closure of periprosthetic paravalvular leaks. J Am Coll Cardiol. 2011;58:2210–7.
4. Sorajja P, Cabalka AK, Hagler DJ, Rihal CS. Long-term follow-up of percutaneous repair of paravalvular prosthetic regurgitation. J Am Coll Cardiol. 2011;58:2218–24.
5. Rihal CS, Sorajja P, Booker JD, Hagler DJ, Cabalka AK. Principles of percutaneous paravalvular leak closure. JACC Cardiovasc Interv. 2012;5:121–30.
6. Swaans MJ, Post MC, Johan van der Ven HA, Heijmen RH, Budts W, ten Berg JM. Transapical treatment of paravalvular leaks in patients with a logistic Euroscore of more than 15%: acute and 3-month outcomes of a "Proof of Concept" study. Catheter Cardiovasc Interv. 2012;79:741–7.
7. Reed GW, Tuzcu EM, Kapadia SR, Krishnaswamy A. Catheter-based closure of paravalvular leak. Expert Rev Cardiovasc Ther. 2014;12(6):681–92.
8. Calvert PA, Northridge DB, Malik IS, Shapiro L, Ludman P, Qureshi SA, et al. Percutaneous device closure of paravalvular leak: combined experience from the United Kingdom and Ireland. Circulation. 2016;134(13):934–44.
9. Cruz-Gonzalez I, Rama-Merchan JC, Calvert PA, Rodríguez-Collado J, Barreiro-Pérez M, Martín-Moreiras J, et al. Percutaneous closure of paravalvular leaks: a systematic review. J Interv Cardiol. 2016;29:382–92.
10. Sanchez-Recalde A, Moreno R, Galeote G, Jimenez-Valero S, Calvo L, Sevillano JH, et al. Immediate and mid-term clinical course after percutaneous closure of paravalvular leakage. Rev Esp Cardiol. 2014;67(8):615–23.
11. Paixao A, Cilingiroglu M. Paravalvular leaks: one size (or shape) doesn't always fit all? Catheter Cardiovasc Interv. 2016;88(4):624–5.
12. Goktekin O, Vatankulu MA, Tasal A, Sönmez O, Başel H, Topuz U, et al. Transcatheter transapical closure of paravalvular mitral and aortic leaks using a new device: first in man experience. Catheter Cardiovasc Interv. 2014;83:308–14.
13. Ercan E, Tengiz I, Turk U, Ozyurtlu F, Alioglu E. A new device for paravalvular leak closure. Case Report. J Geriatr Cardiol. 2015;12:187–8.
14. Goktekin O, Vatankulu MA, Ozhan H, Ay Y, Ergelen M, Tasal A, et al. Early experience of percutaneous paravalvular leak closure using a novel Occlutech occluder. EuroIntervention. 2016;11(10):1195–200.
15. Yildirim A, Goktekin O, Gorgulu S, Norgaz T, Akkaya E, Aydin U, et al. A new specific device in transcatheter prosthetic paravalvular leak closure: a prospective two-center trial. Catheter Cardiovasc Interv. 2016;88(4):618–24.
16. Smolka G, Pysz P, Kozłowski M, Jasiński M, Gocoł R, Roleder T, et al. Transcatheter closure of paravalvular leaks using a paravalvular leak device—a prospective Polish registry. Adv Interv Cardiol. 2016;12(2):128–34.

17. Davidavicius G, Rucinskas K, Drasutiene A, Samalavicius R, Bilkis V, Zakarkaite D, et al. Hybrid approach for transcatheter paravalvular leak closure of mitral prosthesis in high-risk patients through transapical access. J Thorac Cardiovasc Surg. 2014;148:1965–9.
18. Jelnin V, Dudiy Y, Einhorn BN, Kronzon I, Cohen HA, Ruiz CE. Clinical experience with percutaneous left ventricular transapical access for interventions in structural heart defects. A safe access and secure exit. J Am Coll Cardiol Interv. 2011;4:868–74.
19. Smolka G, Pysz P, Jasinski M, Gocoł R, Domaradzki W, Hudziak D, et al. Transapical closure of mitral paravalvular leaks with use of amplatzer vascular plug III. J Invasive Cardiol. 2013;25(10):497–501.

Chapter 5
Echo Guiding During Transcatheter Paravalvular Leak Closure

Piotr Pysz

5.1 Aspects of Echocardiography Imaging Relevant for Transcatheter Paravalvular Leak Closure

5.1.1 Choice of Modality

Transcatheter paravalvular leak closure (TPVLC) is one of the most echo-dependent cardiac structural interventions. During procedures performed under general anesthesia (GE), implementation of transesophageal echocardiography (TEE) is obviously preferable. Nevertheless, the intention to use TEE should not be the only factor motivating the use of GE as TEE probe is usually well tolerated throughout the procedure provided adequate conscious sedation (e.g., intravenous benzodiazepine + fentanyl). Intracardiac echocardiography (ICE) may be considered an alternative to TEE in non-intubated patients but only to a limited extent [1]. With the catheter placed in the right atrium (RA), it is useful for monitoring transseptal puncture, but its so far mainly two-dimensional (2D) nature with only limited three-dimensional (3D) possibilities renders it inferior to real-time (RT) 3D TEE when it comes to navigating within the left atrium (LA).

Paramitral TPVLC is essentially unfeasible without TEE guidance with preferably 3D imaging. First case series demonstrating the superiority of RT-3D TEE over 2D TEE for TPVLC was published in 2010 [2]. RT-3D TEE did not only enable the comprehensive description of shape and size of PVL channel but was also used to identify closely positioned PVLs as separate lesions and then to verify crossing the

Electronic Supplementary Material The online version of this chapter (doi:10.1007/978-981-10-5400-6_5) contains supplementary material, which is available to authorized users.

P. Pysz
Department of Cardiology, Medical University of Silesia, Katowice, Poland
e-mail: piotr.pysz@gmail.com

© Springer Nature Singapore Pte Ltd. 2017
G. Smolka et al. (eds.), *Transcatheter Paravalvular Leak Closure*,
DOI 10.1007/978-981-10-5400-6_5

targeted one. Same authors assessed the effects of TPVLC measuring the reduction of the width and circumferential extent of PVL's orifice.

In some patients with aortic PVL and contraindications to TEE, a procedure monitored solely by TTE may be planned. Finding and crossing an aortic PVL is usually feasible under fluoroscopy but may require repeated aortography. With such approach, echocardiography serves as a tool to monitor for complications (prosthetic discs or mitral chordae impingement, tamponade, etc.) and to assess the effect. As the exact measurement of PVL size may be problematic on TTE, particularly in patient laying on back, previous imaging data is prerequisite (TTE in the lateral position, multi-detector computed tomography—MDCT).

Irrespective of PVL location and imaging technique, it is mandatory to document the amount of pericardial effusion (or lack of it) at baseline to enable reliable monitoring throughout the procedure. Secondly, regardless of previously performed studies, transprosthetic gradient, as well as pulmonary vein inflow pattern in the case of mitral PVL or descending aorta flow in case of aortic PVL, must be recorded again at the beginning of each procedure. Hemodynamic conditions at that time should also be noted (blood pressure, heart rate). Such approach is intended to enhance consistency of TPVLC effect assessment as described below.

Finally, integration of ultrasound images with fluoroscopy for procedural guidance has been reported to further simplify catheter maneuvering during TPVLC [3, 4].

5.1.2   Key Details of PVL Anatomy

A comprehensive description of PVL anatomy is of paramount importance for TPVLC success, whereas the dimensions of observed structures, sometimes on the verge of the resolution reached by echocardiography, often render it an exceptionally difficult task.

The presence of surgical sutures crossing the PVL lumen, though difficult to visualize, may compromise TPVLC outcome unless identified and taken into account while choosing the occluders and technique of their delivery (implantation of several smaller plugs into each of PVL subcompartments vs. implantation of one larger plug to cover the undivided PVL). If stitches themselves are not visible observation of the sewing ring mobility may prove helpful. With large PVLs usually at least small hypermobility ("rocking") of the prosthetic ring can be noted. This is less pronounced with sutures crossing PVL lumen which tend to stabilize the ring—see Movie 5.1 a–f.

Another factor of utmost importance is the identification of the PVL's "narrow neck" if present. Such situation may be caused by the presence of calcium deposits within the PVL channel. These may easily remain unnoticed during 2D TEE examination as they are veiled by highly turbulent flow mapped by color Doppler (CD). RT-3D TEE with CD can enhance visualization of PVL channel shape. It enables sufficient quality of imaging in the vast majority of paramitral leaks but also in some patients with para-aortic leaks, especially those located on the non-coronary and left

Table 5.1 Technical aspects of PVL visualization in RT-3D TEE

Technique	Benefit
Zoom mode + CD acquisition of small volume of tissue containing PVL channel only	Highest possible volume rate
Single-beat acquisition only	Avoidance of stitching artifacts
Multiplanar presentation	Measurements of CSA of VC, minimum and maximum dimensions of VC, channel length

Fig. 5.1 CD-mapped flow across PVL with the identification of true VC (*arrow*)

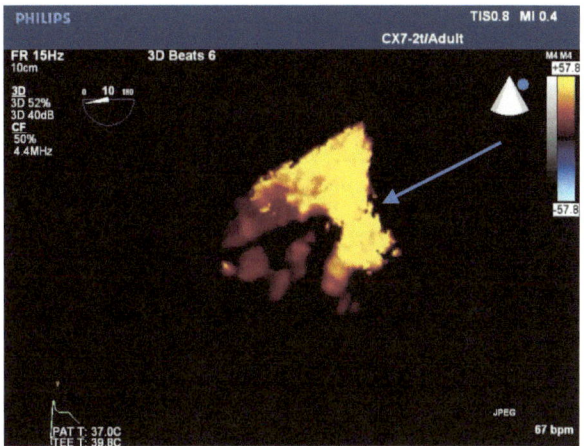

coronary sinuses where no acoustic shadowing by prosthetic valve occurs. Technical aspects of image acquisition are presented in Table 5.1. After the acquisition of the data set, an echo of surrounding tissue may be removed during postprocessing, and, with only CD-mapped flow left, the shape and course of the PVL channel can be appreciated—see Fig. 5.1 and Movie 5.2.

Beside the PVL itself, the appearance of adjoining structures should also be appreciated. The close vicinity of protruding calcium deposits or prosthesis' horns may hinder full expansion of occluding device's discs and thus deteriorate the completeness of PVL sealing, which is particularly relevant should a paravalvular leak device (PLD) be used.

5.1.3 Echo-Driven Choice of Occluding Devices

From a practical standpoint, it is important to allocate the observed PVL into one of two groups presented in Table 5.2. Such approach is intended to choose optimal occluding devices as described in detail in Chaps. 5 and 9 (either Amplatzer Vascular Plug III—AVP III—implanted in multiplug technique or PLD used a single device). For sizing of PVL channel, RT-3D TEE with CD is usually an excellent tool with

Table 5.2 PVL anatomy features relevant for device choice

Suitable for multiplug AVP III	Suitable for single PLD
Irregular/crescent CSA of VC	Round /oval CSA of VC
Channel length >5 mm	Channel length ≤5 mm
Bulks of calcium within channel or surrounding structures that might impede full expansion of discs	No structures potentially impeding disc apposition

previously mentioned limitations related mainly to the location of the lesion. For a multiplug approach, the cross-sectional area (CSA) of the PVL vena contracta (VC) is the key parameter [5]—see Fig. 5.2a, b. Should a PLD be chosen as best anatomy-matched device, minimum and maximum diameters of PVL VC dictate the size of the device without any oversizing [6]—see Fig. 5.3a, b.

5.1.4   Technical Tips

To achieve the best attainable quality of imaging, the most rudimentary technical aspects also need to be taken into account. The first difficulty may be caused by the patient's position during the procedure (horizontal as opposed to left lateral during standard TEE examination). In some patients, it significantly deteriorates the quality of the image. Placing a pillow under patient's right shoulder blade and thus regaining more TEE-friendly heart position within the chest can solve the problem. Long time of procedure may also be of consequence due to gradual drying out of the esophagus. This problem may easily be prevented in most cases by regular use of rubber sheaths for TEE probe amply filled with saline or ultrasound gel.

5.2   Echocardiographic Guidance for Specific PVL Location

Echocardiographic determination of PVL location, discussed in detail in Chap. 4, is pivotal for the choice of the access site. Likewise, the chosen approach for TPVLC poses specific challenges for echocardiography guiding.

5.2.1   Para-aortic Leak: Transvascular Access

In majority of patients, the PVL can usually be easily identified and crossed on fluoroscopy provided the location is known from echo. Thus, in many patients, 2D TEE may be sufficient for TPVLC guiding. Given friendly anatomy, on standard short and long axis (SAX, LAX) views with CD, the CSA of PVL's VC, minimum and maximum dimensions, and the channel length can be measured with satisfying

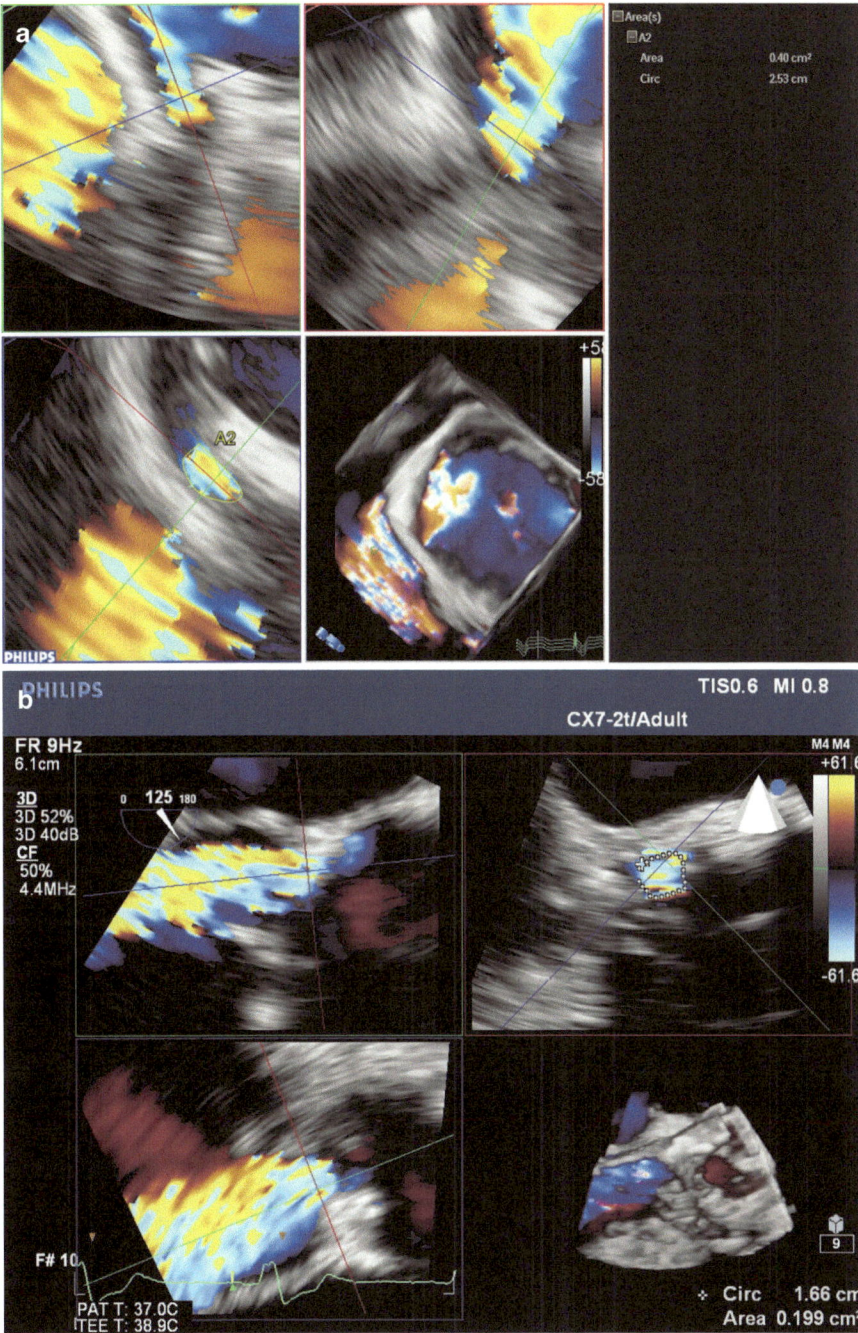

Fig. 5.2 Measurement of cross-sectional area (CSA) of VC in mitral (**a**) and aortic (**b**) PVL

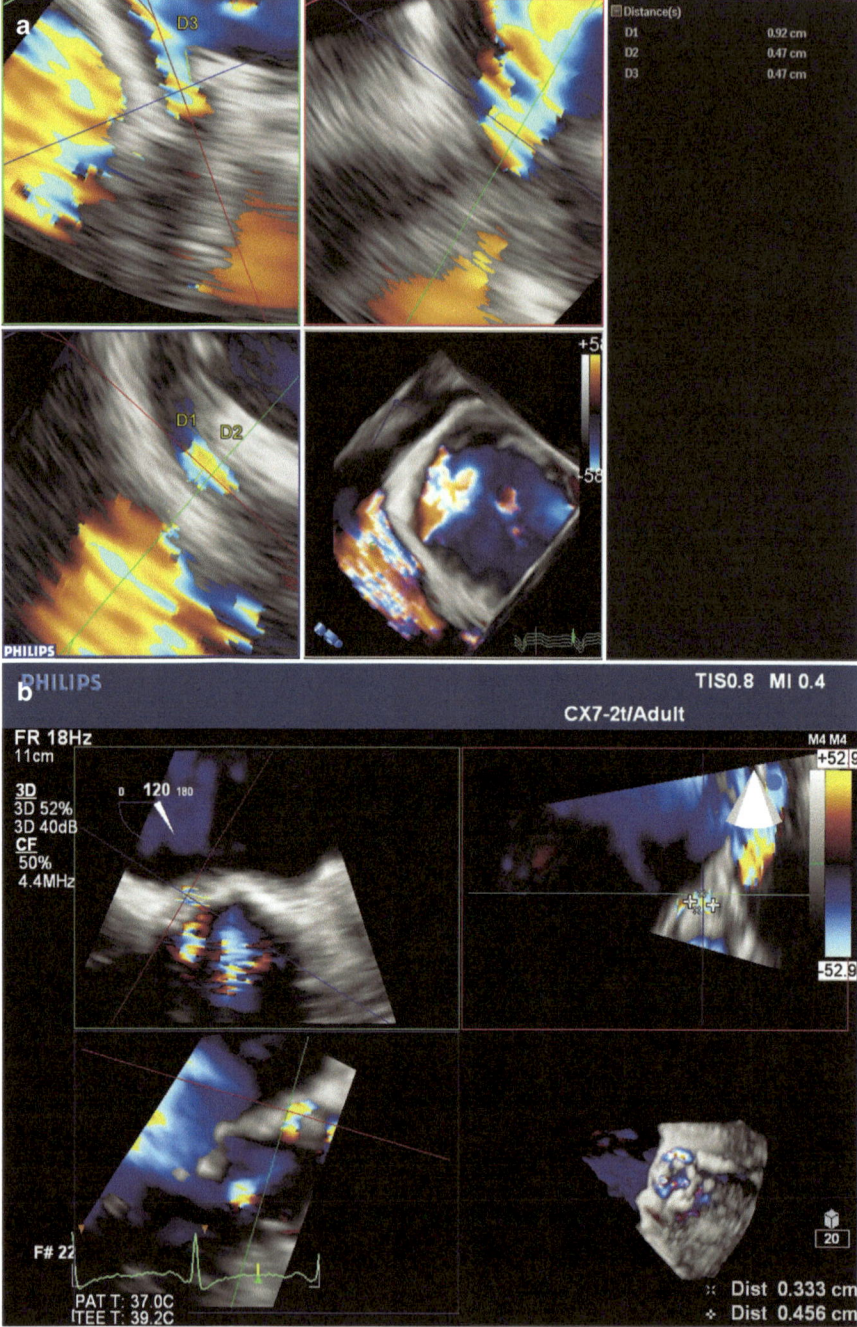

Fig. 5.3 Measurement of maximum and minimum diameters of VC (D1, D2) and length of the channel (D3) in mitral (**a**) and aortic (**b**)

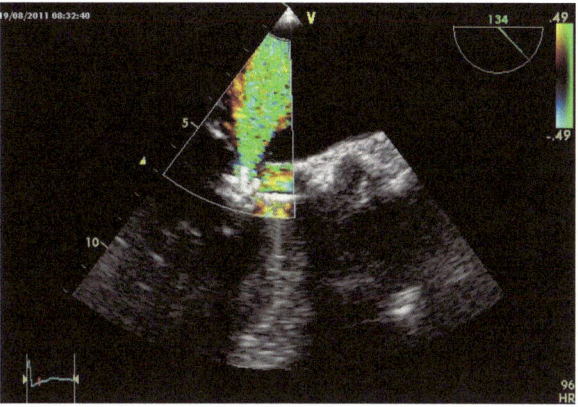

Fig. 5.4 Mitral subvalvular apparatus impingement provoking significant mitral regurgitation noticed during aortic PVL retrograde TPVLC

precision. If the PVL channel is oblique, RT 3D TEE with CD may visualize the course of the channel and identify the true VC dimensions. During TPVLC, performed in a retrograde manner from transfemoral arterial access, constant echo surveillance is needed to identify potential reasons for complications. First, after forming the loop in the left ventricle (LV), the tip of the guidewire may migrate across the mitral valve into LA increasing the risk of tamponade if unobserved. Secondly, retraction of partially opened occluders before their implantation may result in mitral subvalvular apparatus impingement and chordal rupture unless timely identified—Fig. 5.4. If a PLD is used, 3T 3D TEE may visualize the plug's distal disc within the left ventricular outflow tract (LVOT) and thus be helpful in orientating the device properly. After full expansion of occluding devices but before their release, the mobility of prosthetic discs has to be verified, with 2D TEE being usually an excellent tool. Both 2D and 3D TEE are useful for assessment of TPVLC effect as described below.

5.2.2 Paramitral Leak: Transvascular Access

TEE is an excellent tool for transseptal puncture guidance with optimally simultaneous visualization of interatrial septum in two orthogonal planes, an option offered by 3D TEE probes. The definition of optimal puncture site varies according to PVL location and planned strategy. For PVL channels located in anterolateral aspects of the mitral ring, a direct access may be the easiest route with optimal puncture site being middle to high. In PVLs located in posteromedial aspects of the ring, two possibilities may be considered. First, a steerable catheter can be used with relatively high puncture site (to accommodate the curve of the sheath within the LA). Alternatively, forming a loop within the LA can optimize the angulation of the catheter tip, which in turn enhances the chance of crossing (relatively low puncture site to gain enough space within LA for loop formation)—see Fig. 5.5.

Fig. 5.5 A loop formed with a catheter in LA—note the alignment enhancing the chance of successful crossing of PVL

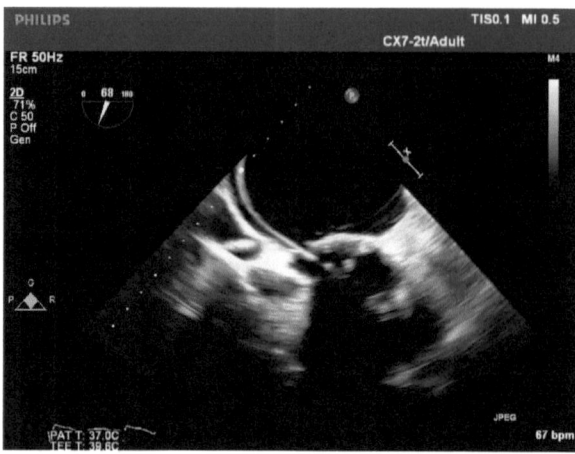

Regardless of strategy, RT 3D TEE with volume rendering (VR) visualization is a perfect tool for piloting the operator toward the PVL orifice. For this purpose live single-beat imaging is used starting with full volume for general navigation. Once the tip of the catheter is positioned in the vicinity of PVL and pointing toward its orifice, the 3D VR image should be switched to zoom mode. Thus, the direction of guidewire extension can be visualized and angulation of the catheter optimized if needed—see Movie 5.3. Once the guidewire enters the LV, both 2D and 3D are useful for confirmation of crossing the PVL and not the prosthetic valve. Next, the formation of wire loop within the LV should be monitored by echo to reduce the risk of LV perforation. Acoustic shadowing by mitral prosthesis may sometimes be a major hindrance that can be evaded by moving to transgastric views. In some cases, the guidewire is advanced into the ascending aorta for better support, and then the degree of transient iatrogenic aortic regurgitation needs to be observed (usually irrelevant). During the implantation of occluding devices, constant attention has to be paid to the mobility of prosthetic discs. In some patients, RT 3D TEE with VR enables visualization of distal PLD disc within the LV and may help to optimally orientate the device. As with aortic PVLs, preservation of prosthetic disc mobility has to be confirmed after full expansion of the plug(s) but before their release.

5.2.3 *Paratricuspid Leak: Transvascular Access*

The experience with tricuspid PVLs is obviously much smaller than with those located in left heart chambers. Typically, deep transesophageal probe position results in optimal visualization of tricuspid prosthesis ring with either four-chamber or SAX views. RT 3D TEE VR imaging is also possible and utilized, with quality less spectacular than within the LA but sufficient for navigation.

5.2.4 Transapical Access: Lateral Minithoracotomy

As a first step TTE may be helpful for choosing optimal intercostal space for performing a thoracotomy. Once that is completed, TEE biplane views of the LV apex with surgeon's finger pressing from outside identify the best puncture site. Echo guiding of the catheter within the LV is usually much compromised by acoustic shadowing in transesophageal views. As mentioned before, transgastric views may circumvent the shadowing, but then the PVL is usually poorly visible except for posterior location. Nevertheless, information gained from echo may support the fluoroscopy guidance by defining the relations between PVL location and structures visible on X-ray images like prosthesis' horns or hinges. After crossing the PVL, TEE becomes the fundamental tool again with excellent visualization of occluders within the LA—Fig. 5.6. With no shadowing from delivery systems (sometimes present during transseptal procedures), echocardiography gives perfect control of plug(s)' orientation, the level of implantation, and the efficacy of sealing.

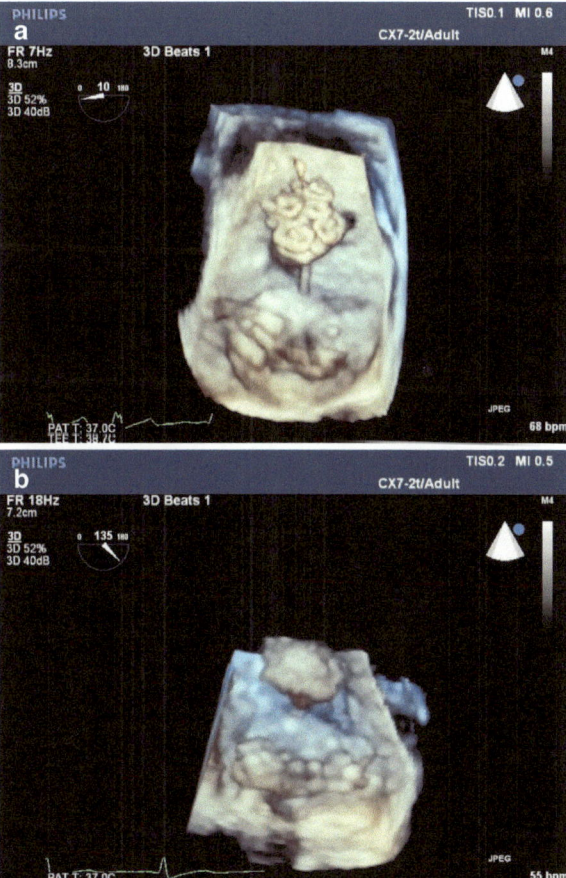

Fig. 5.6 RT 3D TEE VR image of AVP III (**a**, multiplug technique) and PLD (**b**) devices before implantation during mitral TPVLC with transapical access

5.2.5 Transapical Access: Direct Percutaneous Puncture

Percutaneous left ventricular transapical access, among other structural interventions, is also utilized for TPVLC [7]. It requires additional preprocedural imaging to optimize the puncture site and to avoid injury to lung tissue, coronaries, and papillary muscles. For this purpose, MDCT is an excellent tool, also used as an overlay on the live fluoroscopic image during the procedure. Further echocardiographic guiding following percutaneous apical puncture is similar as with transapical access with lateral thoracotomy. This approach may also involve device closure of apical access site to prevent bleeding.

5.3 Assessment of TPVLC Acute Effect

Ensuring comparable hemodynamics conditions at baseline and then during the assessment of TPVLC effect is a prerequisite. This predominantly involves maintaining similar blood pressure by administering intravenous fluids or catecholamines in a patient-tailored manner.

Reduction of CD-mapped flow is the first and most rudimentary indicator of TPVLC efficacy—if completely eliminated it obviously proves excellent result—Fig. 5.7. The presence of residual flow requires further analysis. Provided sufficient echocardiography image quality, comparison of VC CSA by RT 3D TEE with CD after TPLVC to that at baseline is the most direct approach to quantify the PVL reduction.

Secondly, complementary indicators such as reduction of transprosthetic flow velocity gradient (expected after eliminating the volume overload caused by PVL), normalization of flow pattern in pulmonary veins (mitral PVL), and descending aorta (aortic PVL) should be looked for. Importantly, for all three parameters, the

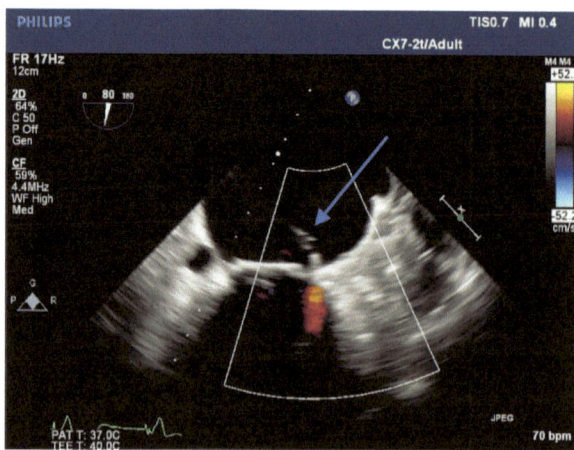

Fig. 5.7 Complete obliteration of mitral PVL documented by CD-mapping before release of PLD (*arrow* pointing at delivery cable)

measurements should be taken in exactly same views pre- and postprocedurally to ensure identical ultrasound beam alignment.

Other manifestations of altered hemodynamic state may also indirectly hint at good TPVLC result. Instant appearance of spontaneous echo contrast (SEC) in usually dilated LA suggests a significant reduction of backflow after mitral TVPLC—Movie 5.4. In patients with stentless aortic prostheses implanted in subcoronary position, the PVL drains the so-called dead space between the native aortic sinuses and scarf of the prosthetic valve. After successful TPVLC instant clotting of the "dead space" can be observed—Movie 5.5. Lastly, the direction of shunt across PFO, if present, may also prove the hemodynamic changes following meaningful PVL reduction as shown in the case of tricuspid PVL—Fig. 5.8.

Finally, should this multifactorial echocardiography analysis produce unclear or contradictory findings, one should remember about direct hemodynamic parameters such as LA pressure in mitral and diastolic pressure in aortic PVLs (easily available during TPLVC).

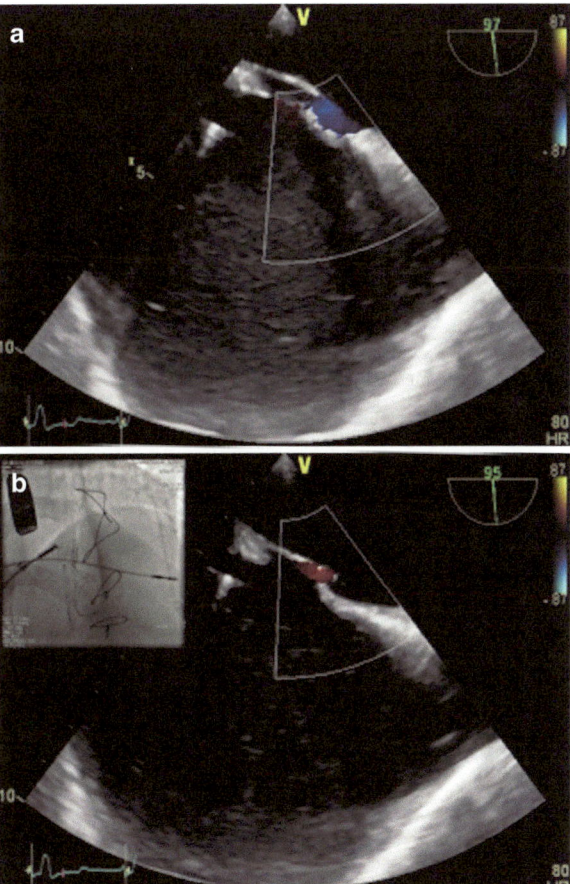

Fig. 5.8 Change of shunting direction across PFO following tricuspid TPVLC (**a**, baseline; **b**, after PLD implantation)

References

1. Krishnaswamy A, Kapadia SR, Tuzcu EM. Percutaneous paravalvular leak closure—imaging, techniques and outcomes. Circ J. 2013;77(1):19–27.
2. Biner S, Kar S, Siegel RJ, et al. Value of color Doppler three-dimensional transesophageal echocardiography in the percutaneous closure of mitral prosthesis paravalvular leak. Am J Cardiol. 2010;105(7):984–9.
3. Balzer J, Zeus T, Hellhammer K, et al. Initial clinical experience using the EchoNavigator(®)-system during structural heart disease interventions. World J Cardiol. 2015;7(9):562–70.
4. Biaggi P, Fernandez-Golfín C, Hahn R, et al. Hybrid imaging during transcatheter structural heart interventions. Curr Cardiovasc Imaging Rep. 2015;8(9):33.
5. Smolka G, Pysz P, Jasiński M, et al. Multiplug paravalvular leak closure using Amplatzer Vascular Plugs III: a prospective registry. Catheter Cardiovasc Interv. 2016;87(3):478–87.
6. Smolka G, Pysz P, Kozłowski M, et al. Transcatheter closure of paravalvular leaks using a paravalvular leak device—a prospective Polish registry. Postepy Kardiol Interwencyjnej. 2016;12(2):128–34.
7. Jelnin V, Dudiy Y, Einhorn BN, et al. Clinical experience with percutaneous left ventricular transapical access for interventions in structural heart defects a safe access and secure exit. JACC Cardiovasc Interv. 2011;4(8):868–74.

Chapter 6
Fusion Imaging for Paravalvular Leak Closure

Tilak K.R. Pasala, Vladimir Jelnin, Itzhak Kronzon, and Carlos E. Ruiz

6.1   Introduction

Paravalvular leak (PVL) is a well-recognized complication after heart valve surgery and transcatheter valve replacement [1, 2]. Historically, repeat open-heart surgery has been the mainstay of treatment for paravalvular leaks [1]. However, recent advances in transcatheter therapies have made percutaneous closure of PVLs a less invasive and safe alternative, especially in those at high risk for repeat surgery. Percutaneous repair of PVLs can be associated with considerable complexity and is advised to be performed at experienced centers [3]. These procedures are heavily reliant on various imaging modalities for pre-procedural planning and intraprocedural guidance. Traditionally, these procedures were guided by 2-dimensional (2D) echocardiographic and fluoroscopic guidance to project complex 3D anatomy. Understandably, this posed challenges for acquiring spatial information that is needed to perform these procedures effectively and safely. The advent of echocardiography and computed tomography angiography (CTA) into 3D and 4D visualization and post-processing technology has allowed a more comprehensive understanding of the anatomy and better intraprocedural guidance. However, individual modalities like fluoroscopy and echocardiography provide different information of the anatomy and are presented separately. It can be challenging for operators to piece together these parallel information simultaneously. The integration of CTA with fluoroscopy (CTA-fluoroscopy fusion) and echocardiography with fluoroscopy (echo-fluoroscopy fusion) in the catheterization laboratory allows operators to overcome many of the challenges posed when these imaging modalities are used

T.K.R. Pasala • V. Jelnin • C.E. Ruiz, MD, PhD, FACC, FESC, MSCAI (✉)
Structural and Congenital Heart Center, Joseph M. Sanzari Children's Hospital,
Hackensack University Medical Center, Hackensack, NJ, USA
e-mail: CRuiz@StructuralHeartCenter.org

I. Kronzon
Lenox Hill Hospital and Vascular Institute of New York, New York, NY, USA

© Springer Nature Singapore Pte Ltd. 2017
G. Smolka et al. (eds.), *Transcatheter Paravalvular Leak Closure*,
DOI 10.1007/978-981-10-5400-6_6

individually. Merging relevant information from different imaging modalities on to a composite image, commonly referred to as fusion imaging, has been shown to improve efficacy and safety and reduce the requirement of radiation, contrast, and procedural time [4]. More importantly, fusion imaging provides more accurate intraprocedural guidance when approaching PVL closure.

6.2 Challenges During Closure of Paravalvular Leak

Complex structural heart disease procedures like PVL closure can be highly demanding for the multidisciplinary team (interventional cardiologist, cardiac surgeon, imaging specialist, etc.) performing it. All members of the team are required to have a comprehensive understanding of the anatomy, continuous intraprocedural recognition, and spatial understanding of the relationships between catheters and wires to cardiac structures. More importantly, a successful and safe procedure relies highly on the effective second to second communication between the interventionalist and imaging specialist. Some of the miscommunication is due to limitations of the various imaging modalities. Fluoroscopy is inherently limited to provide 3D spatial information and does poor characterization of non-radiopaque structures. Echocardiography on the other hand is limited by window availability and the inability to detect the position of the catheters and wires. Additionally, the orientation of the images from various modalities is different. For example, rotating the c-arm can project the same cardiac structures differently. This can add extra demand on the interventionalist to communicate and orient to echocardiography simultaneously and vice versa. The real-time integration of the imaging modalities that provide volumetric datasets, which fluoroscopy cannot provide, would offset some of the above limitations. Fusion imaging provides a more rapid recognition and orientation of cardiac structures facilitating an improved communication between members of the multidisciplinary team.

6.3 Image Acquisition and Preprocedural Planning for PVL

6.3.1 Image Acquisition—Computed Tomography Angiography

The procedural planning with CT requires high-quality source CT data; hence, expertise in acquisition of CT images is important. High-quality images can be generated with high spatial and temporal resolution using helical CT, multi-row detectors (MDCT), and ECG gating. CTA data is acquired in helical mode with simultaneous recording in ECG, then multiple phases (from 10 up to 20) of cardiac cycle are reconstructed using retrospective ECG triggering protocol. Prospective gating with acquisition during a selected single phase of the cardiac cycle has lesser radiation dose and can be typically used for younger patients. Nonionic contrast

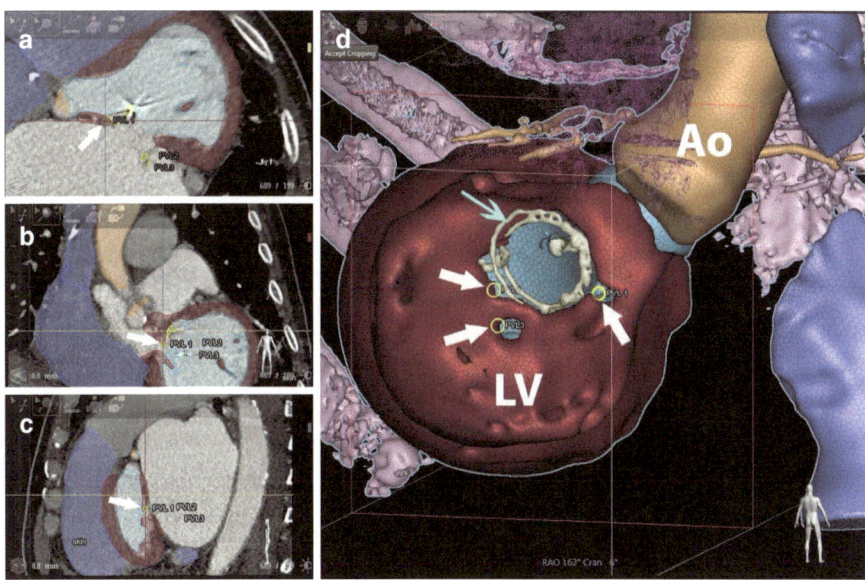

Fig. 6.1 Windows on the left (**a–c**) demonstrate the process of identification of different cardiac structures by applying the designated color mesh on the standard anatomical planes (axial, sagittal, and coronal) [5]. A three-dimensional model with markers placed on the location of paravalvular leaks (**d**, *white arrows*) and metallic valve (**d**, *blue arrow*) are shown

media injection at 60–90 mL (adjusted for patient size and renal function) at the rate of 5–6 mL/s via antecubital vein is usually utilized, and image acquisition is timed for peak contrast concentration in the left ventricle.

A 3D model of the heart structures can be generated by automatic segmentation of the CTA data using tools in HeartNavigator (Philips Healthcare, Best, The Netherlands) (Fig. 6.1). The system allows options to manually adjust the contour of the heart structures, add new structures, change opacity, apply cut planes, perform measurements, subtract irrelevant structures, and place markers.

6.3.2   Image Acquisition—Echocardiography

The acquisition of 2D and 3D datasets is an important aspect of using fusion imaging for PVL closure. Acquisition is done live at the time of the procedure which can then be fused with live fluoroscopy. We describe it in this section for continuation. For acquiring high-quality and relevant images, the 3D fully sampled matrix array TEE transducer (3D–MTEE) has become integral [6]. It has approximately 2500 elements, in contrast to the 64 elements in the multiplane TEE probes [7]. With this transducer several 3D echo protocols or imaging modes are routinely used; (1) The "xPlane mode" displays two images, one is the reference 2D image and the second a rotated view of the reference image which can be manipulated (rotated or tilted) (2). The "real-time narrow-angle mode" displays a narrow pyramidal dataset with excellent spatial and temporal resolution; however cardiac structures cannot be fully imaged (3). The "3D–zoom mode" displays a wider sector view of the region of interest which can be rotated in all directions. This mode is useful for guiding catheters/wires and visualizing devices. However, it suffers in temporal resolution (4). In the "full-volume ECG-gated mode," a full-volume 3D dataset and 3D full-volume color Doppler are obtained over four heartbeats and stitched together. This can then be manipulated online or offline in dedicated software [6]. The full-volume mode is useful to identify the location of the PVLs but may be limited by poor spatial resolution and stitch artifact [8–10]. With the use of the above modes, PVL can be visualized in multiple views; e.g., the mitral PVL can be visualized both from the surgical view and the ventricular view, thus guiding catheters and wires. The color Doppler helps in locating PVLs pre- and interprocedurally. All the above modes can be used in the echo-fluoroscopy fusion imaging.

6.3.3 Identification of PVL and Virtual Planning

The value of tailoring preprocedural planning for PVL closure for each patient cannot be understated. It includes evaluation of the anatomical location, number, extent, course, severity, and surrounding structures of PVL. The post-processing of CTA data is performed as described above facilitating annotation of relevant structures during or prior to the procedure.

MDCT combined with echocardiography can determine the size, shape, course, and the surrounding cardiac structures of the PVLs [11, 12]. (Figs. 6.1d, b) In addition, valuable information on the prosthetic valve structure (pannus formation, leaflet thickening, adjacent calcification, pseudoaneurysm, etc.) and function (abnormal leaflet mobility) can be obtained [13, 14]. Two-dimensional and 3D color Doppler helps with localizing the PVL and when fused with fluoroscopy can help with precise steering of catheters and wires.

Virtual planning can be done by post-processing pre-acquired CT data (Fig. 6.2). A virtual line joining the skin entry, LV entry, and PVL can be drawn which then can be fused with fluoroscopy. In addition, virtual implantation of various devices can be simulated on the model which may help the interventionalist in predicting the size and the number of devices that may be required (Fig. 6.2c).

6.4 Principles of Fusion Imaging

Fusion image can be defined as a composite synergistic image where the most relevant information datasets from two or more different imaging modalities are combined in a comparable scale and displayed as a new image. Fusion imaging does not provide new information, but it enhances it in a more relevant manner. Fusion

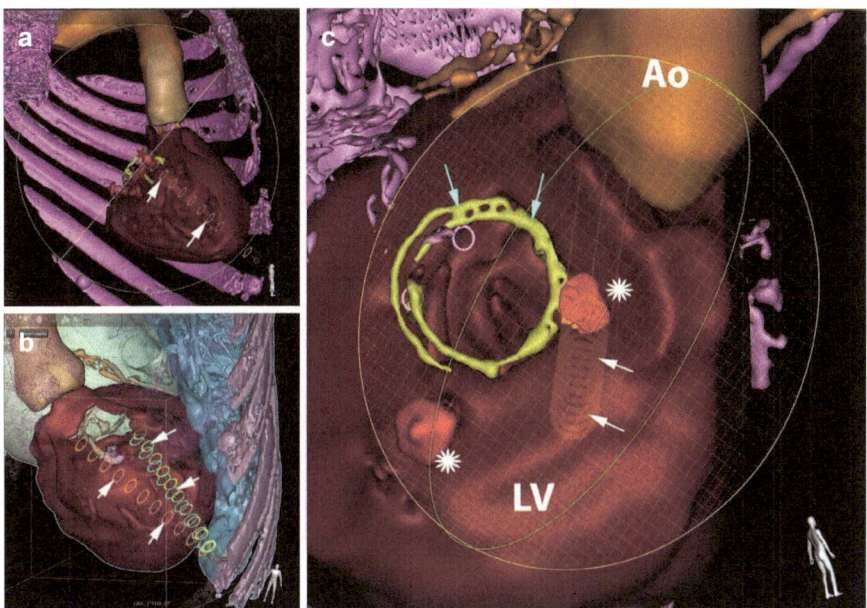

Fig. 6.2 Virtual PVL closure planning. The safe path from the skin puncture site to the location of PVLs at different locations can be virtually placed (**a**, **b**, *white arrows*). On the 3D segmented model, virtual models of the Amplatzer vascular plugs (**c**, *asterisk*) are placed to examine the possible size and interactions with surrounding structures including prosthetic valve (**c**, *blue arrows*)

imaging is being used in multiple specialties of medicine. One such example is the single photon emission computed tomography (SPECT) and CT fusion which is used for evaluation of coronary disease, localizing infection (white cell infection imaging), orthopedic/sports injury imaging (bone scan SPECT-CT), etc. The ability to merge these images provides a more accurate identification of the anatomical location and extent (from CT) of the abnormalities highlighted on SPECT nuclear medicine scans. In performing complex structural heart procedures like PVL closure, merging and projection of a live or preprocessed image (typically echocardiograph or CTA) over another image (typically live fluoroscopy) is used (Fig. 6.3).

6.4.1 Echocardiography-Fluoroscopy Fusion

The initial step of the fusion process is co-registration of two distinct images, which is to orient one image (images from echocardiography) to another image (fluoroscopy). Echo-fluoroscopy fusion relies on real-time co-registration which involves spatially orienting echocardiographic image to match fluoroscopic image. This can be automatically performed by the EchoNavigator® system which uses TEE probe localization and calibration algorithm for co-registration (Fig. 6.4). It relies on

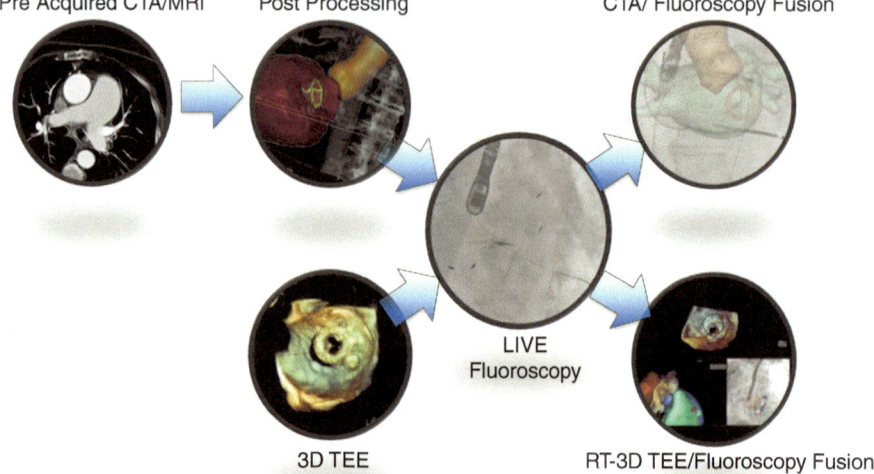

Fig. 6.3 Schematic of fusion imaging for PVL closure. Pre-acquired CTA/MRI data (post-processed) and 3D TEE data are fused with live fluoroscopy for CTA-fluoroscopy fusion and echo-fluoroscopy fusion

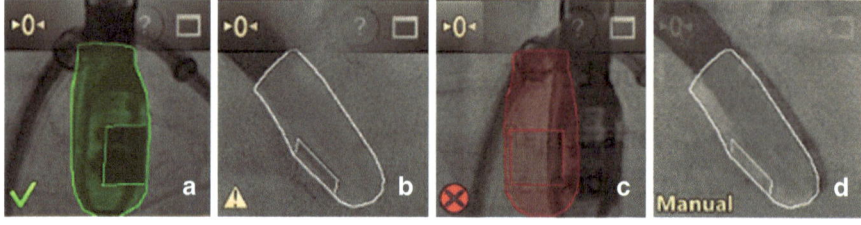

Fig. 6.4 TEE probe registration is performed automatically when the probe is in the X-ray field of view by stepping on the X-ray pedal. When registration is successful, a check mark is visible, and the probe is displayed in *green* (**a**); transparent, registration timed out (**b**); *red*, unsuccessful (**c**); in special cases registration could be performed manually (**d**) by adjusting the contour position till it becomes *green*

rapid, automated identification of TEE probe tip during live fluoroscopy. The TEE transducer is housed in a plastic shell and has a characteristic signature on X-ray projection, which changes on probe position and angulation predictably [15].

It is able to automatically tract the position and the direction of the TEE probe and overlay chosen 3D echo imaging mode on the fluoroscopic image [16]. Subsequently, the system tracks and follows the rotation of the C-arm and synchronizes the echo image with fluoroscopic image. Several different echo views can be displayed by the system (Fig. 6.5); (1) The echo view shows images that are seen by the echocardiographer (2). The C-arm view shows the TEE field of view (i.e., echo cone) as a purple sector along with corresponding TEE images. (3) The free view allows additional post-processing capability like reorientation, cropping in any plane of interest [15].

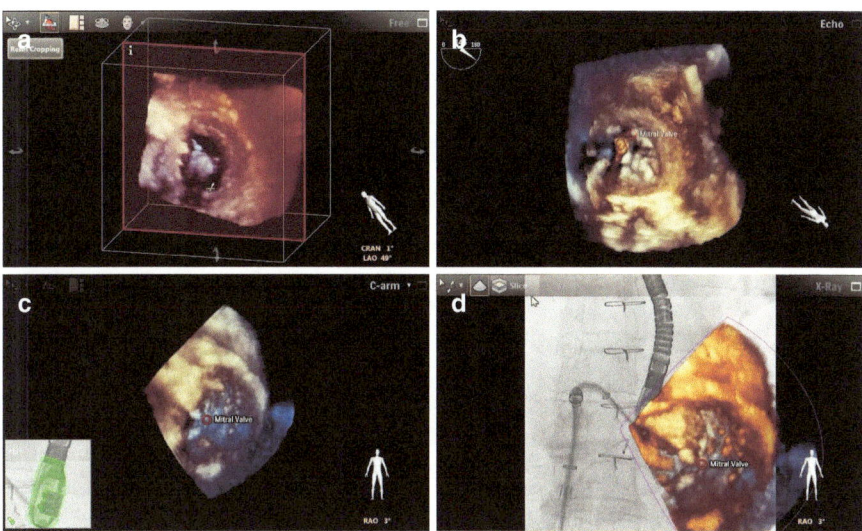

Fig. 6.5 Work windows of EchoNavigator. (**a**) The free view where the 3D image can be manipulated with active cut plane tool (*red plane*) allowing cutting the 3D reconstructed volume and free 360° rotation. (**b**) The standard 3D view controlled by 3D TEE operator. (**c**) A 3D–view orientation defined by the position of TEE probe (*green*) is shown. (**d**) The C-arm view which shows the fusion of the 3D TEE volume (*purple sector*) over the live fluoroscopy

Additionally, annotation markers can be placed at the site of PVL based on 3D TEE zoom and 3D color Doppler. The system automatically translates this marker on the fluoroscopic image and fixes it regardless of subsequent TEE probe position (Fig. 6.5c, d).

6.4.2   CTA-Fluoroscopy Fusion

Co-registration between CTA and fluoroscopy can be achieved by using existent radiopaque markers (i.e., prosthetic valve metal frame, pacemaker wires, calcification, etc.) or by registering with contrast aortography (Fig. 6.6). Once the co-registration is achieved, the overlaid CTA image and markers move with real-time fluoroscopy providing a 3D orientation of the cardiac structures during procedures.

6.5   Intraprocedural Guidance for PVL

6.5.1   Access

Access to closure of PVLs is chosen dependent on the location of the PVL and operator experience. Multiple approaches have been described including antegrade transseptal from the inferior vena cava, retrograde transapical through the left ventricular puncture, and retrograde transaortic from the aorta crossing the aortic valve [17].

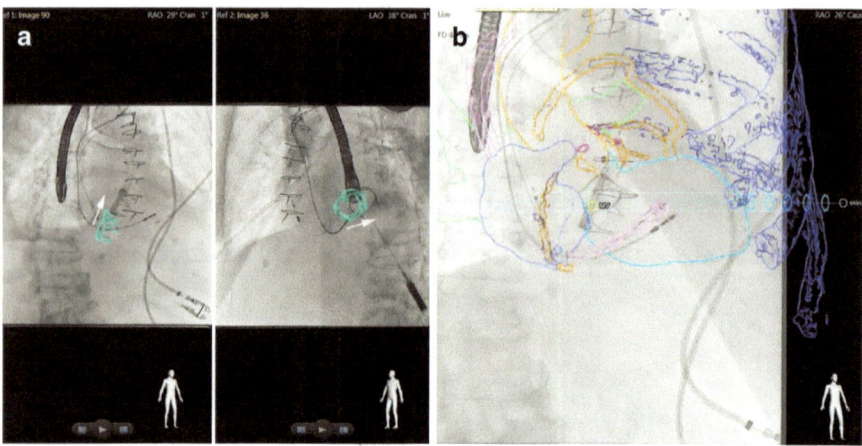

Fig. 6.6 Registration of CT segmentation over the live fluoroscopy. Registration is achieved by manually adjusting the segmented prosthetic valve (**a**, *blue color*) over the prosthetic valve visible on fluoroscopy. Two orthogonal planes at least 20° apart (**a**: RAO 29° and LAO 38°) are used to move the segmented prosthetic valve to overlay the position seen on the fluoroscopy (**a**). After the desired positioning is achieved and accepted, the 3D model of the cardiac structures with target markers placed during preprocedural planning will follow the C-arm position and will help to guide the intervention by displaying the precise location of the defects in 3D space (**b**)

6.5.1.1 Transseptal

Transseptal puncture is commonly used for PVL closure, and a quick but safe puncture of the interatrial septum is the first step. The RT-3D TEE-fluoroscopy fusion offers tools for locating the optimal puncture site by placing markers (Fig. 6.7a) on TEE that can be translated to fluoroscopy. Biplane or 3D TEE can be fused with fluoroscopy aiding a more control puncture and advancement of needle/catheter (Fig. 6.7b).

6.5.1.2 Transapical

Transapical access can be safe in the hands of experienced operators. With the addition of CTA-fluoroscopy fusion, the actual transapical puncture site can be guided as close to preplanned puncture site as possible. It also helps to maintain a safe distance from the lungs and left anterior descending artery (Figs. 6.2a, b, and 6.8) [4, 18]. Closing of the transapical access is done by deploying an AVP II device through sheath used for access. Overlaying the borders of LV on fluoroscopy along with contrast injection helps in confirming the position of the device.

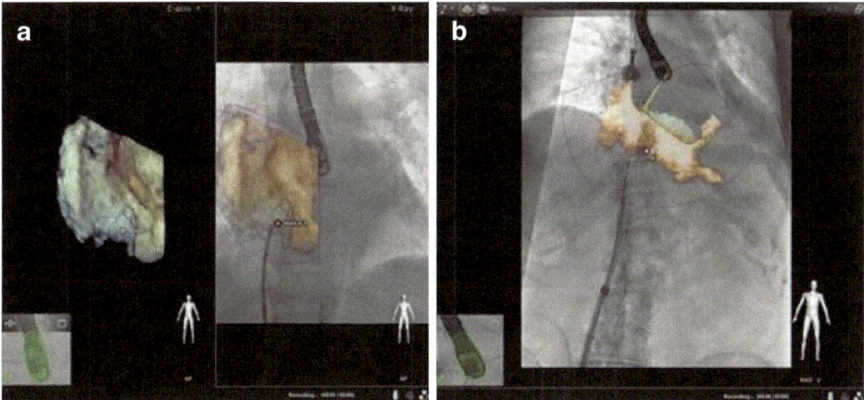

Fig. 6.7 Echo-fluoroscopy fusion for transseptal guidance

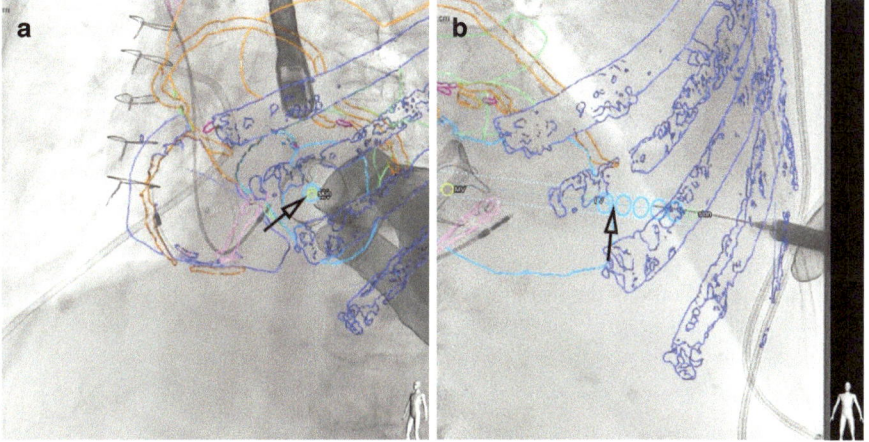

Fig. 6.8 CTA-fluoroscopy fusion guidance for transapical puncture. On two different views (**a**, LAO, and **b**, AP view), the "safe path" (*blue*) which is joining the puncture site to the paravalvular leak (*yellow marker*) is overlaid on the top of fluoroscopy. Operator can rotate the C-arm to an angle where the "safe path" is seen as a circle (**a**, *black arrow*). This allows for steering the needle in the direction of the PVL more precisely

6.5.2 Crossing PVL and Device Placement

With the use of RT-3D TEE-fluoroscopy fusion, steering of catheters and wires is easier as they can be delineated with combination of the fluoroscopy and echo images. Additionally, color Doppler shows the precise location of PVL which aids

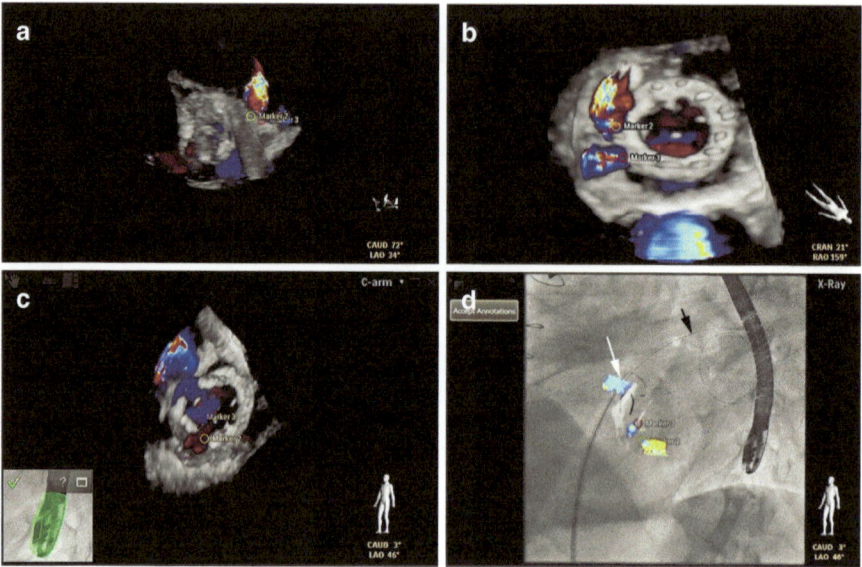

Fig. 6.9 TEE-fluoroscopy fusion using color Doppler mode. Paravalvular leaks are identified by the location of the regurgitant jets on color Doppler (**a–c**; *markers*). The fusion of color Doppler over fluoroscopy helps in crossing the PVLs (**d**, *white arrow*). An Inoue wire (Toray Industries, Inc.) is noted in the left atrium (*black arrow*)

in crossing of wires and deployment of devices. RT-3D TEE fluoroscopy fusion can compensate for some of the limitations of CTA-fluoroscopy fusion by providing live guidance which is helpful in crossing the PVLs (Figs. 6.9, 6.10, 6.11, and 6.12).

6.5.3   PVL Post-Transcatheter Aortic Valve Replacement

With the advent of transcatheter aortic valve replacement (TAVR) and poor outcomes with PVL post-TAVR, closing PVL may be of significance [19]. Techniques of PVL closure in prosthetic valves using fusion imaging can be translated to post-TAVR PLVs.

6.6   Limitations of Fusion Imaging

Few limitations of fusion imaging should be highlighted. First, when there is significant motion of the cardiac structures, the static annotations of CTA-fluoroscopy fusion can make it challenging. Moving the C-arm to a more coaxial angle or using the color Doppler fusion may offset this limitation. Second, drift in annotation

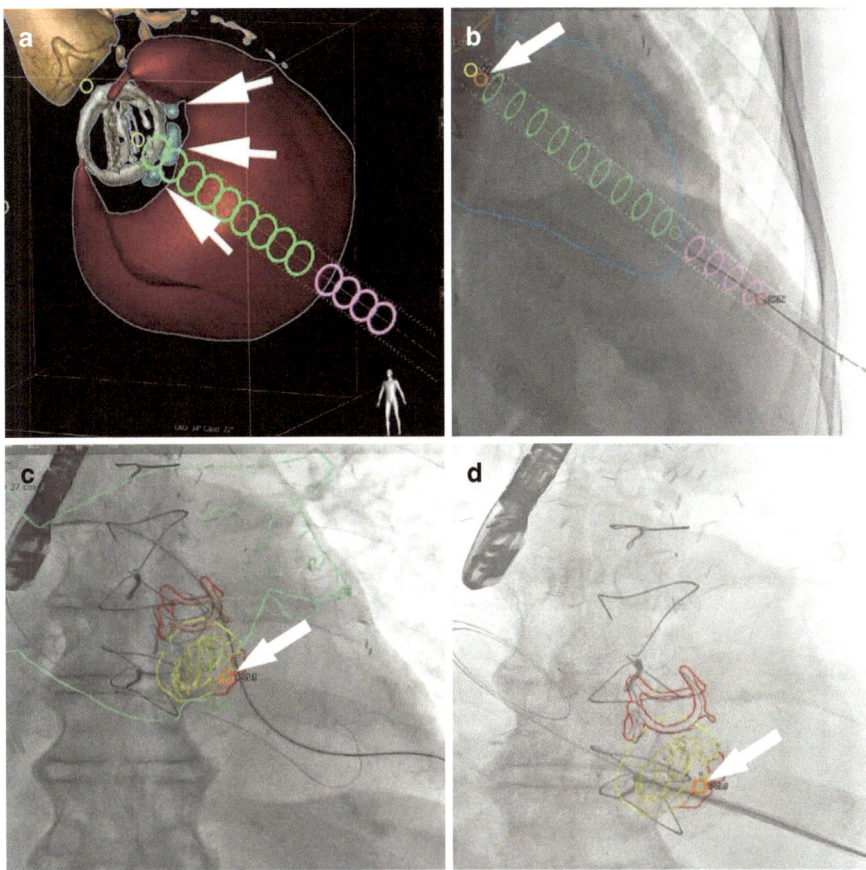

Fig. 6.10 Intraprocedural guidance for PVL closure with CTA-fluoroscopy fusion. (**a**) Planning the procedure by using 3D segmentation of cardiac structures, marking the PVL (*white arrows*) and the safe path for transapical puncture. (**b**) Guidance of transapical puncture, white arrow pointing to PVL marker (*orange color*) placed during planning. (**c**) Demonstrates the guidance of CTA-fluoroscopy fusion for crossing the PVL. (**d**) A closure device is seen in the first PVL, when catheter with safety wire is placed in the second PVL

points can occur where markers on echo may drift causing registration error [15]. Third, fusion imaging is a growing technology, and the availability of this technology is limited to a few centers. The lack of widespread availability could be due to incompatibility with existent fluoroscopic systems, slow adoption of newer technology, and exposure of this technology among interventional cardiologists. Fourth, there is need for further evidence on clinical endpoints with the use of this technology. So far there is no randomized trial comparing this technology with standard imaging [20]. Lastly, the initial high cost of this technology may prohibit some centers from acquiring it.

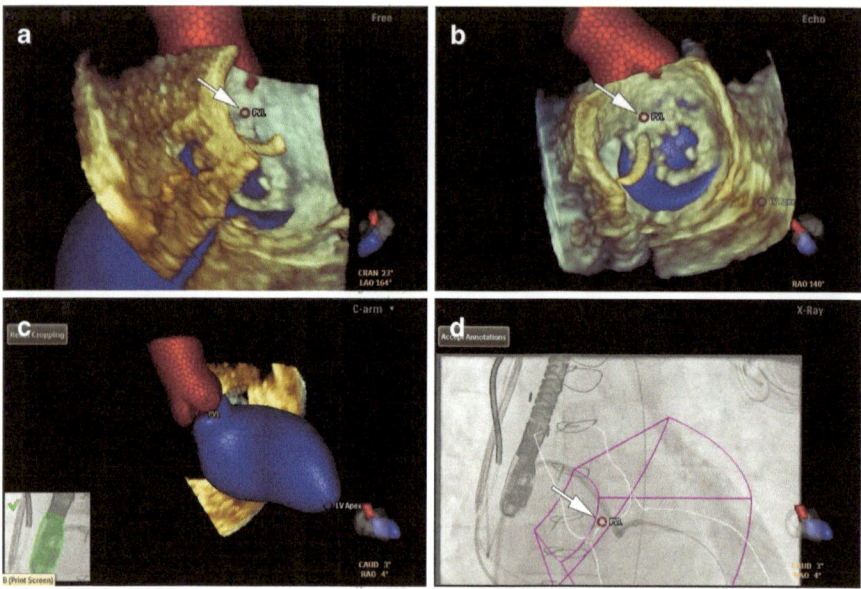

Fig. 6.11 TEE-fluoroscopy fusion for antegrade transseptal PVL closure. Catheter is seen crossing the PVL (*white arrow*)

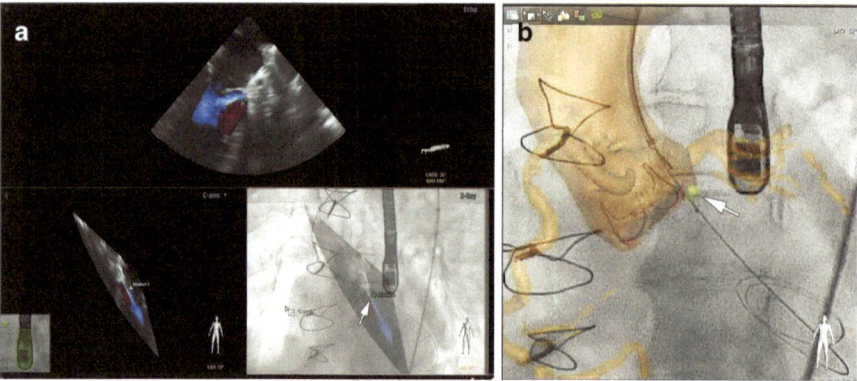

Fig. 6.12 TEE-fluoroscopy fusion during aortic PVL closure. (**a**) Color Doppler demonstrates a significant regurgitant flow through the PVL. (**b**) CTA-fluoroscopy fusion of a 3D model with marked PVL (*yellow marker*) is overlaid over the fluoroscopy

6.7   Future of Fusion Imaging

The field of percutaneous structural heart disease intervention is progressing rapidly into a new era. Fusion imaging is positioned to provide real-time and more accurate guidance for complex procedures. First, fusion of live echo and CTA fusion may decrease the use of live fluoroscopy thus decreasing overall radiation dose and contrast use. Second, with the advancement in MRI technology, MRI-fluoroscopy fusion may improve spatial resolution and soft tissue characterization in addition to decreasing the overall radiation. Third, simulating and predicting the final device deployment by defining soft tissue characteristics (i.e., tensile strength) may be challenging but a useful capability. Fourth, the automation of some of the steps of preprocedural planning may encourage the adoption of this technology. As the imaging technology advances, the future looks bright and it is imperative for interventionalists doing these procedures to be mindful of the advancements taking place in this field.

6.8   Summary

PVL is a challenging disease associated with poor outcomes. Closure of PVL is a complex procedure dependent on comprehensive understanding of the 3D anatomy, imaging modalities, and prompt communication between the interventionalist and imaging specialist. Fusion imaging with echo-fluoroscopy fusion and CTA-fluoroscopy fusion can provide additional guidance at various steps of the PVL closure. More importantly, it can improve the communication between the members of the heart team. This technology is still in early stages, and additional studies are needed to assess its impact on clinical outcomes. Operators interested in PVL closure procedures should invest the time in training in fusion imaging as it has tremendous potential to be a game changer in complex structural heart disease procedures like PVL closure.

References

1. Akins CW, Bitondo JM, Hilgenberg AD, et al. Early and late results of the surgical correction of cardiac prosthetic paravalvular leaks. J Heart Valve Dis. 2005;14:792–9. Discussion 799800 2005;14 SRC—GoogleScholar:792–9.
2. Smith CR, Leon MB, Mack MJ, et al. Transcatheter versus surgical aortic-valve replacement in high-risk patients. N Engl J Med. 2011;364:2187–98.
3. Nishimura RA, Otto CM, Bonow RO, et al. 2014 AHA/ACC guideline for the Management of Patients with Valvular Heart Disease: a report of the American College of Cardiology/American Heart Association task force on practice guidelines. J Am Coll Cardiol. 2014;63:e57–e185.
4. Kliger C, Jelnin V, Sharma S, et al. CT angiography-fluoroscopy fusion imaging for percutaneous transapical access. JACC Cardiovasc Imaging. 2014;7:169–77.
5. Waechter I, Kneser R, Korosoglou G, et al. Patient specific models for planning and guidance of minimally invasive aortic valve implantation. Med Image Comput Comput Assist Interv. 2010;13:526–33.
6. Vegas A, Meineri M. Core review: three-dimensional transesophageal echocardiography is a major advance for intraoperative clinical management of patients undergoing cardiac surgery: a core review. Anesth Analg. 2010;110:1548–73.

7. Sugeng L, Shernan SK, Salgo IS, et al. Live 3-dimensional transesophageal echocardiography: initial experience using the fully-sampled matrix array probe. J Am Coll Cardiol. 2008;52:446–9.

8. Lang RM, Badano LP, Tsang W, et al. EAE/ASE recommendations for image acquisition and display using three-dimensional echocardiography. J Am Soc Echocardiogr. 2012;25:3–46.

9. Hahn RT, Abraham T, Adams MS, et al. Guidelines for performing a comprehensive transesophageal echocardiographic examination: recommendations from the American Society of Echocardiography and the Society of Cardiovascular Anesthesiologists. J Am Soc Echocardiogr. 2013;26:921–64.

10. Perk G, Lang RM, Garcia-Fernandez MA, et al. Use of real time three-dimensional transesophageal echocardiography in intracardiac catheter based interventions. J Am Soc Echocardiogr. 2009;22:865–82.

11. Lesser JR, Han BK, Newell M, Schwartz RS, Pedersen W, Sorajja P. Use of cardiac CT angiography to assist in the diagnosis and treatment of aortic prosthetic paravalvular leak: a practical guide. J Cardiovasc Comput Tomogr. 2014;9:159–64.

12. Ruiz CE, Jelnin V, Kronzon I, et al. Clinical outcomes in patients undergoing percutaneous closure of periprosthetic paravalvular leaks. J Am Coll Cardiol. 2011;58:2210–7.

13. Chenot F, Montant P, Goffinet C, et al. Evaluation of anatomic valve opening and leaflet morphology in aortic valve bioprosthesis by using multidetector CT: comparison with transthoracic echocardiography. Radiology. 2010;255:377–85.

14. Habets J, Mali WP, Budde RP. Multidetector CT angiography in evaluation of prosthetic heart valve dysfunction. Radiographics. 2012;32:1893–905.

15. Thaden JJ, Sanon S, Geske JB, et al. Echocardiographic and fluoroscopic fusion imaging for procedural guidance: an overview and early clinical experience. J Am Soc Echocardiogr. 2016;29:503–12.

16. Gao G, Penney G, Ma Y, et al. Registration of 3D trans-esophageal echocardiography to X-ray fluoroscopy using image-based probe tracking. Med Image Anal. 2012;16:38–49.

17. Jelnin V, Kliger C, Zucchetta F, Ruiz CE. Use of computed tomography to guide mitral interventions. Interv Cardiol Clin. 2016;5:33–43.

18. Jelnin V, Dudiy Y, Einhorn BN, Kronzon I, Cohen HA, Ruiz CE. Clinical experience with percutaneous left ventricular transapical access for interventions in structural heart defects a safe access and secure exit. JACC Cardiovasc Interv. 2011;4:868–74.

19. Genereux P, Head SJ, Hahn R, et al. Paravalvular leak after transcatheter aortic valve replacement: the new Achilles' heel? A comprehensive review of the literature. J Am Coll Cardiol. 2013;61:1125–36.

20. Biaggi P, Fernandez-Golfin C, Hahn R, Corti R. Hybrid imaging during transcatheter structural heart interventions. Curr Cardiovasc Imaging Rep. 2015;8:33.

Chapter 7
Transcatheter Closure of Paravalvular Leaks: Procedural Aspects

Grzegorz Smolka and Wojciech Wojakowski

Transcatheter closure (TPLVC) has become a safe, feasible, and efficient approach in the treatment of patients with heart failure and hemolysis related to paravalvular leaks (PVLs) on surgical valve prostheses. It has been accepted as an alternative to redoing surgery in patients with a high risk of reoperation and favorable anatomy in the American Heart Association/American College of Cardiology 2014 Guidelines for the Management of Patients with Valvular Heart Disease [1, 2] as a class IIa indication (level of evidence B).

For many years, due to lack of a dedicated device, TPLVC was done with the off-label use of plugs approved for the treatment of congenital heart disease (atrial septal defect, ventricular septal defect, patent ductus arteriosus). Since 2015 a dedicated device has been approved in Europe; however it is not available in the USA. Accumulating clinical experience with TPLVC showed that the majority of operators use two types of devices: Amplatzer Vascular Plug-type devices (St. Jude Structural Division of Abbott, USA), in particular AVP II and III, and the dedicated plug [paravalvular leak device (PLD), Occlutech, Switzerland]. The diversity of PVL anatomy and localization requires specific training and a customized approach regarding procedural techniques on top of experience in the treatment of structural heart diseases.

G. Smolka (✉) • W. Wojakowski
Department of Cardiology and Structural Heart Diseases, Medical University of Silesia, Katowice, Poland
e-mail: gsmolka@me.com

© Springer Nature Singapore Pte Ltd. 2017   105
G. Smolka et al. (eds.), *Transcatheter Paravalvular Leak Closure*,
DOI 10.1007/978-981-10-5400-6_7

7.1 Choice of Devices

Regardless of the location of the leak and access, there is a toolbox of wires, sheaths, and catheters which should be available for every procedure.

Guidewires: standard coronary 190 and 300 cm guidewires, 0.035″ 260 and 300 cm wires with a range of stiffness (regular, extra stiff, super stiff) and hydrophilic 0.035″ wires. For the creation of arteriovenous loop and removal of embolized devices, the 25–35 mm snares should be available. A range of delivery sheaths is of key importance. Dedicated sheaths recommended by specific device manufacturers can be used. However, PVL often requires a tailored approach using peripheral vascular sheaths, as the dedicated sheaths are sometimes too short for aortic PVLs in particular. Most practical are peripheral guiding sheaths with a hydrophilic coating of the distal part. Braided sheaths are less susceptible to lumen loss due to the tortuosity of the PVL channel. Coronary sheathless guide catheters may be used as well; however, their elasticity at the distal end might be disadvantageous in case of the retraction and reposition of the plug, which can produce deformation of the distal edge.

The steerable sheaths available in different curves and lengths offer additional maneuverability and support, especially in the case of navigation in the atrium.

7.2 Procedural Approaches

7.2.1 Aortic PVL

The easiest access to PVL located on the prosthetic aortic valve is retrograde through the femoral artery [3]. Usually, the delivery system is ≤8F, and in the case of multi-plug approach, bifemoral access can be used. The vascular closure device is frequently used in particular in patients with a mechanical prosthetic valve on oral anticoagulants. For larger sheaths, preclosure with suture-based systems is preferable. In the case of advanced aortoiliac atherosclerosis, brachial artery access can be used because it accommodates all necessary sheath sizes. In a small number of selected cases, a direct aortic approach is also an option. Radial access has the potential advantage of reduction of complications associated with bleeding, but also significant limitations related to the maximum size of the delivery system, the length of the sheath, and the increased mechanical force required to navigate the sheath through the artery and PVL channel [4]. Several published cases described the antegrade approach with a septal puncture and mitral valve crossing; however, such an approach has limited indications.

Preprocedural planning is based on transthoracic (TTE) or transesophageal echocardiography (TOE) which allows identification of sinus of Valsalva in which the PVL is located and an initial estimation of its size. Due to the frequent supra-annular position of the prosthetic valve and oblique track of the PVL channel,

Fig. 7.1 Aortic paravalvular leak located in the left coronary sinus. Fluoroscopic projection perpendicular to the plane of the prosthetic valve. Telescopic system with 6F AL1 guide catheter (above the PVL) and 5F long JR diagnostic catheter in the left ventricle

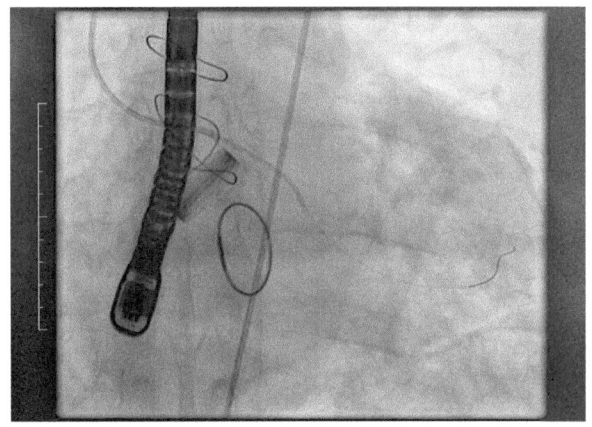

accurate sizing is often challenging. Intraprocedural, the choice of the fluoroscopic projection is crucial, with the preferred one perpendicular to the plane of the ring. PVL should be projected laterally to the perimeter of the prosthetic valve (Fig. 7.1). The next step is navigation with the catheters to identify the PVL channel. A telescopic (mother-and-child) system using a 6F coronary guiding catheter and 125 cm 5F diagnostic catheter (Fig. 7.1) seems to be most useful. The choice of the guiding catheter depends on the location of the PVL. For leaks located in the left coronary sinus, the best option is AL1 or AL2 depending on the aortic root size. After navigating the tip of the catheter into the left coronary sinus and below the ostium of the left main coronary artery, a diagnostic JR is used to engage the PVL channel. For PVL located in the non-coronary or right coronary sinus, the preferred guide catheter would be multipurpose or Judkins right. Such an approach provides improved steerability, and gentle contrast injections allow for PVL localization. A regular 0.014″ coronary guidewire is used for the crossing of the defect, and a Y connector allows for correction of the catheter position using contrast injections. PVL is then crossed with a 5F diagnostic catheter and 6F guide. This step can be difficult due to the oblique axis of the leak, serpiginous track, or calcifications.

Several techniques can facilitate the crossing:

- Increased support by means of a second 0.014″ coronary wire or 0.018″ extra support wire (e.g., V-18 Control Wire, Boston Scientific).
- If a 5F diagnostic catheter is used to cross the PVL, it might be used to introduce 0.035–0.038″ wire to increase support for crossing with a 6F guide (if it is used for plug delivery) or an alternative delivery sheath.
- Use of a long 300 cm coronary guide, withdrawal of the 5F diagnostic catheter, and dilatation of the channel with 2.5 mm balloon. Such an approach may provide gradual tapering of the tip of the guide catheter and modify the calcifications within the PVL, but does not usually increase the diameter of the leak. Also, inflation of the balloon can provide valuable information on the anatomy of the leak, and use of the TOE with a color Doppler can improve the sizing of

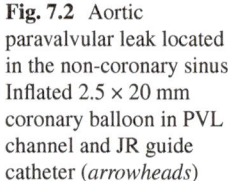

Fig. 7.2 Aortic paravalvular leak located in the non-coronary sinus. Inflated 2.5 × 20 mm coronary balloon in PVL channel and JR guide catheter (*arrowheads*)

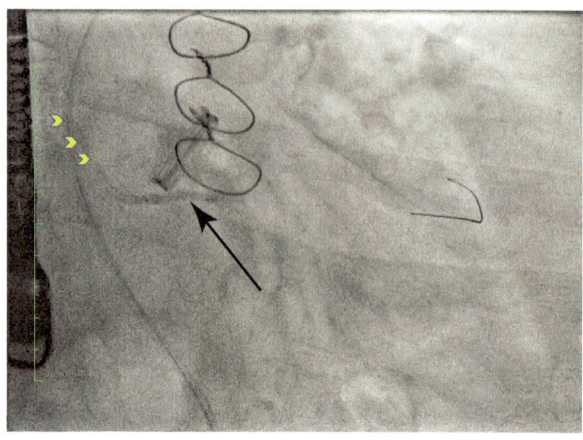

the leak. Use of the partially inflated balloon facilitates the crossing with a delivery catheter or sheath (Fig. 7.2). This technique is not useful, however, when the PVL consists of multiple channels separated by surgical sutures.

In the majority of cases, these techniques allow for the crossing of the PVL with a delivery sheath or catheter sized according to the type and size of the device and in the case of a multiplug approach to their number.

Several approaches can accomplish the delivery of the plug(s):

1. Use of a single PLD device

    The design of the paravalvular leak device (PLD, Occlutech, Switzerland) was discussed in previous chapter and previously published [5, 6]. It is particularly suitable for PVL devices of a length shorter than 4–5 mm. In terms of the implantation technique, the following issues are important:

    - Rectangular occluders have two radiopaque markers in the middle of the longer axis, and these should be maximally separated to allow alignment with the long axis of the leak.
    - The occluder is connected to the delivery cable by the bulb and socket-type connection, so the torque of the delivery cable does not translate into the rotation of the plug. Proper orientation of the device can be achieved by the withdrawal of the proximal disc into the delivery sheath and its torque. In cases in which this is not possible, the plug can be advanced into the left ventricle and withdrawn slowly. After several attempts, the left ventricle wall movement may produce the proper alignment of the device.
    - The distal part of the delivery cable consists of the stiff metallic tubular element. In cases of an oblique PLV track and in patients with a small diameter of the aorta at the level of sinuses of Valsalva and sinotubular junction, this feature of the device may increase the procedural complexity.
    - The W-type PLD should not be oversized. In fact, a small undersizing might be of advantage. The occluder should be sized based on the nominal size. Notably, the size given for the W-type occluders refers to the waist, not the proximal and distal discs [6].

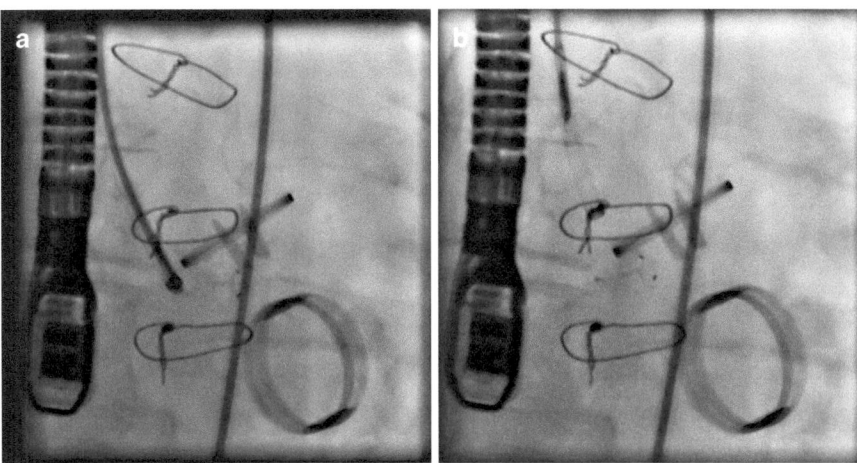

Fig. 7.3 Panel (**a**) The 6 × 3W PLD occluder in the left ventricle with two separated radiopaque markers indicating the proper orientation in relation the long axis of the leak. Panel (**b**) Implanted PLD occluder. Please note that the axis of the PVL is almost perpendicular to the annulus

Exemplary Case
In a patient with PVL located in the non-coronary sinus, the strategy was to implant a single rectangular 6 × 3 mm W-type PLD occluder. The PVL was crossed with a 110 cm 7F delivery sheath, and the occluder was introduced into the left ventricle. It was impossible to rotate the occluder due to the tension and bend of the delivery sheath. The sheath was withdrawn into the PVL channel, and the occluder loosely protruded into the ventricle allowing for spontaneous rotation with the wall movement. This technique led to self-orientation of the plug which subsequently was withdrawn into the sheath in a manner in which the proximal disc was retracted into the sheath just distal to the end of the PVL (Fig. 7.3a). Subsequently, the proximal disc was deployed on the aortic side of the PVL by the withdrawal of the sheath. After the stability test (pull and push technique) and fluoroscopic evaluation of the movement of the prosthetic valve discs and assessment of the residual leak by TOE, the PLD was released. The final result is shown in Fig. 7.3b.

2. Sequential implantation of single/multiple AVP III occluders

AVP III plugs can be implanted individually or using a multiplug technique [7–9]. In the first instance, a larger size of the plug is necessary. It is associated with the increased length of the plugs which, in the case of shorter channels, can lead to excessive overhanging of the distal discs and possibly collision with the disc of the valvular prosthesis. Another solution is to implant two or more smaller and shorter plugs into the single PVL channel which leads to improved filling of the leak channel.

Exemplary Procedure
Figure 7.4 shows the implantation of two 6 × 3 mm AVP III occluders through a single 7F delivery sheath. One occluder was fully deployed in the left ventricle, while the second was partially (proximal disc) withdrawn into the sheath. The

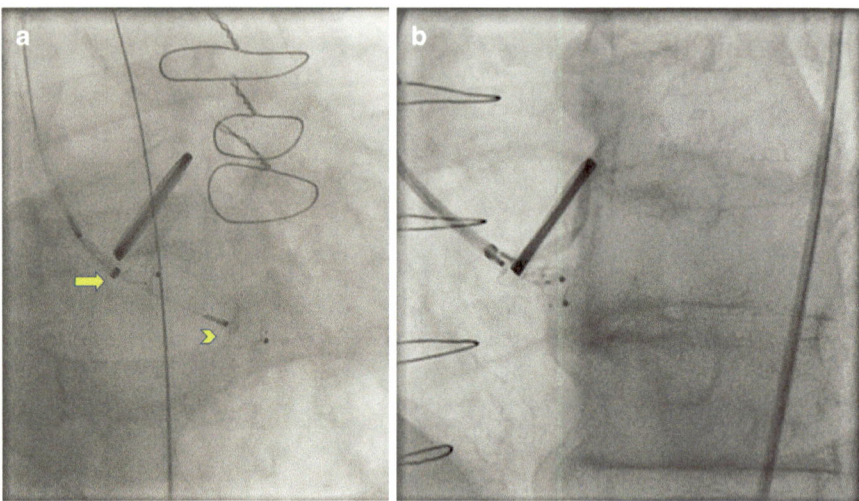

Fig. 7.4 Panel (**a**) Step one: first AVP III plug (*arrow*) just before the deployment of the proximal (aortic) disc, second plug (*arrowhead*) in the left ventricle. Panel (**b**) Step two: both occluders deployed, before release from delivery cable

sheath was withdrawn into the implantation position on the aortic side of the leak (Fig. 7.4a). The first occluder was fully deployed. As the next step, the sheath was forwarded toward the proximal disc acting as a support preventing it from being withdrawn from the PVL channel. The second occluder was pulled through the leak providing full sealing. The final effect is shown in Fig. 7.4b.

Such a technique is an alternative to the simultaneous deployment of two occluders through a single delivery sheath. It provides better tracking control and lessens the risk of pulling occluders out of the channel. It is technically more demanding, however. Also, it is important to understand that the plug is connected to the delivery cable by a screw, so there is a potential risk that the plugs might spontaneously unscrew if the plugs move loosely with the left ventricle before implantation.

In case there is a need to implant more than two AVP III plugs, several approaches are possible:

Figure 7.5 shows the simultaneous implantation of three 6 × 3 mm AVP III plugs through the 8F delivery sheath in a patient with large PVL located in the non-coronary cusp. The size of the leak and lack of calcifications allowed for the easy passage of the delivery sheath. Distal discs of all three occluders were simultaneously exposed from the sheath in the ventricle and were pulled into contact with the prosthetic valve. Through withdrawal of the sheath, the occluders were deployed in the proper position. In such cases, the sequential deployment of the plugs is also feasible as shown in Fig. 7.6. The first two occluders are deployed simultaneously (Fig. 7.6a), followed by delivery of the third plug (Fig. 7.6b).

Fig. 7.5 Multiplug
technique. Simultaneous
deployment of three AVP
III plugs into the PVL
related to aortic
bioprosthesis

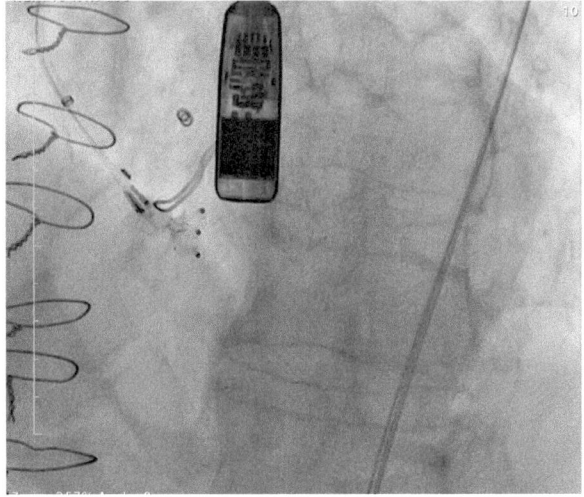

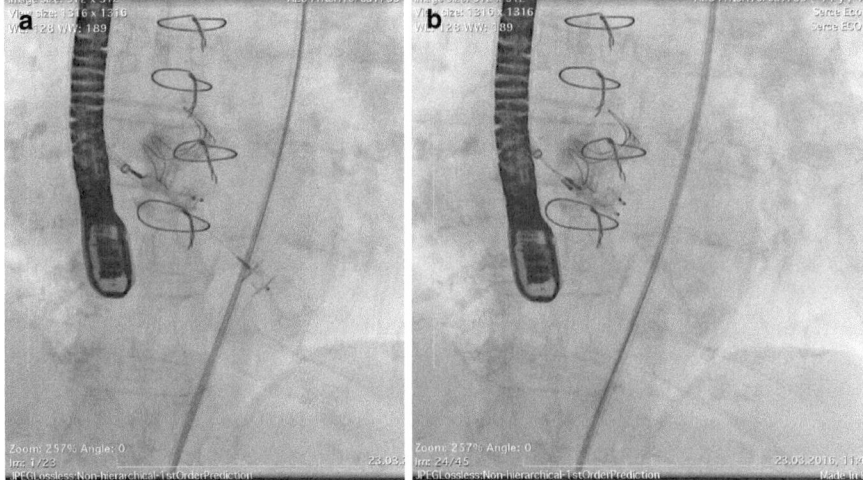

Fig. 7.6 Multiplug technique. Panel (**a**) simultaneous deployment of two AVP III plugs and third
still in the left ventricle. Panel (**b**) Third plug pulled into PVL

In the case of very large leaks, the multiplug technique may require two delivery
sheaths introduced through two arterial punctures. As shown in Fig. 7.7, a large leak
on the aortic bioprosthesis was achieved by implanting four AVP III plugs using two
long sheaths with two occluders each. Such an approach allows for the stable
deployment of all four occluders, evaluation of the PVL sealing, and plug stability
by means of TOE and fluoroscopy before release.

Additional occluders can also be implanted in cases in which, after the implantation of a single AVP III, the PVL is still significant (e.g., underestimation of PVL size).

Fig. 7.7 Multiplug
technique. Four AVP III
implanted using two
parallel delivery sheaths

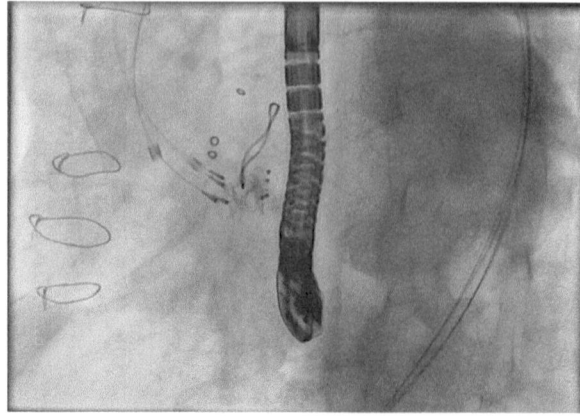

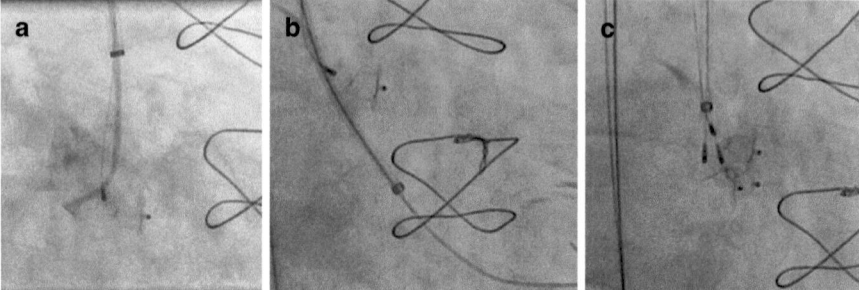

Fig. 7.8 Multiplug technique. Panel (**a**) AVP III deployed, JR 5F catheter in the delivery sheath. Panel (**b**) Deployed plug still connected to the delivery cable. Delivery sheath recrossing the PVL channel. Panel (**c**) Three AVP III plugs prior to release (two implanted through the delivery sheath)

To minimize the risk of embolizing the first occluder, the PVL is recrossed with a 5F JR catheter through the delivery sheath (Fig. 7.8a) followed by the guidewire. Usually, 260–300 cm stiff 0.035–0.038″ exchange-length guidewire is used to withdraw the delivery sheath leaving the delivery wire of the first occluder outside. Subsequently, the sheath is reintroduced over the stiff wire parallel to the delivery wire. This does not usually produce substantial bleeding at the access site because of the small profile of the wire (Fig. 7.8b). The delivery sheath allows for the implantation of the additional occluder(s) to achieve complete sealing of the leak as shown in Fig. 7.8c.

7.2.2   Mitral PVL

Mitral PVLs can be repaired percutaneously using antegrade (transseptal) or retrograde (crossing of the aortic valve) approaches. The choice depends primarily on the location of the leak and the operator's preference. In our experience, the following rules apply:

1. The transseptal approach is preferred for a PVL located anteriorly or anterolaterally (in the proximity of LAA).
2. The transseptal approach can be used but is more challenging for a PVL located in the septal side of the prosthetic valve.
3. PVLs located posteriorly and laterally can pose some difficulties using this approach.

The advantage of the transseptal approach is that it is safe when large diameter delivery systems are used. Also, it provides superior imaging of the prosthetic valve using RT-3D TOE when visualizing from the atrial side of the leak, when compared to transapical and retrograde approaches. In our hands, the retrograde approach may be considered as an alternative to transapical when the septum cannot be crossed safely (thickened, surgical patch, occluder) or there are pathologies in the inferior vena cava (thrombus).

7.2.2.1 Septal Crossing and Delivery of the Guiding Sheath

Septal puncture should be carefully preplanned using the echo and/or CT imaging. The height and anteroposterior location of the puncture site are crucial for successful access to the PVL.

After a septal puncture and heparin dose, navigation in the left atrium may be done using two methods: (1) telescopic system using the 6F guide and 5F diagnostic catheters and (2) steerable sheath (e.g., Agilis). The 2D and 3D TOE guide navigation usually allow the positioning of the catheter tip above the PLV entrance. The choice of coronary catheters depends on the operator's experience, the location of the leaks (loop for septal location vs. direct access for lateral), and the size of the left atrium.

The operator must prepare for difficulties with the puncture and crossing of the IAS in this population of patients. The bailout strategies include:

1. Sharper transseptal needles (e.g., XS version of St. Jude needles)
2. Use of the stiff end of coronary guidewire introduced through the transseptal needle
3. Use of electrocoagulation

Such techniques facilitate the crossing but might increase the risk of perforation, so the periprocedural imaging and choice of the puncture site are crucial.

If, after the crossing, the sheath cannot be advanced, the puncture can be dilated with a 4.0–6.0 mm angioplasty balloon after the crossing of the septum with the needle and the introduction of the coronary guidewire.

7.3   Leaks Located in the Proximity of IAS

Such a PVL can be approached using the loop created by two coronary catheters or directly with a steerable sheath.

Direct access requires distance between the puncture site and PVL to provide space for the curvature of catheters. With the standard transfemoral puncture, it creates an acute angle between the end of the delivery sheath and the inflow of the PVL, which makes crossing difficult. This can compromise the stability of the plugs which cross the PVL in the non-perpendicular plane. Such a case is shown in Fig. 7.9 with two AVP III plugs deployed and thus being pulled toward the leak. The acute angle between the long axis of the delivery catheter and PVL plane is even more challenging when a multiplug approach is used. In particular, the final step of the plug positioning requires stability of the entire delivery system. An example of such a scenario with four AVP III plugs is shown in Fig. 7.10.

In the case of difficulties, an alternative approach would be to perform sequential plug deployment as shown in Fig. 7.11. The safety wire left across the leak when

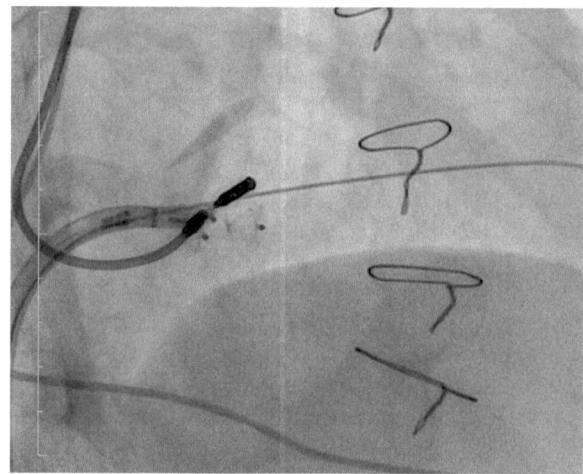

Fig. 7.9 Multiplug technique. Mitral PVL located in the proximity of the intra-atrial septum closed with three AVP III plugs. Two occluders are deployed, and the third is in the left ventricle. The acute angle between the long axis of the leak and the delivery sheath poses a technical challenge

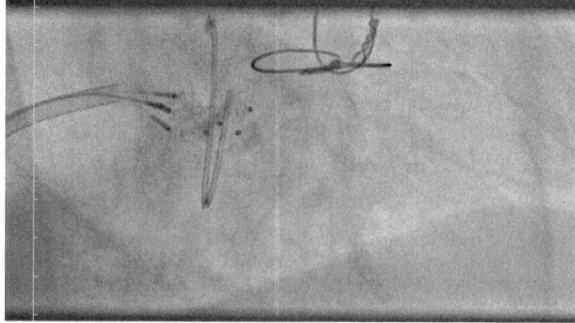

Fig. 7.10 Multiplug technique. Simultaneous implantation of four AVP III plugs into the mitral PVL using single sheath. The mitral bioprosthesis is hardly visible. The tricuspid valvuloplasty ring overlaps the mitral valve prosthesis

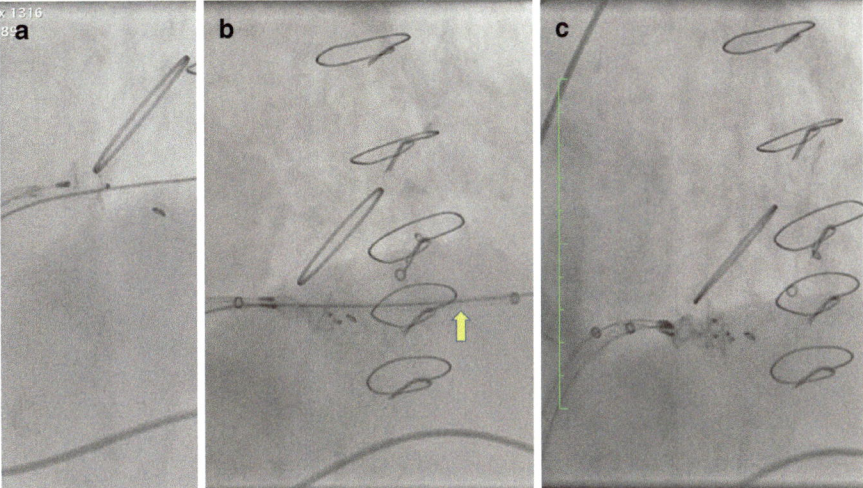

Fig. 7.11 Mitral PLV located in the proximity of the intra-atrial septum. Panel (**a**) After the crossing of the leak with the telescopic system (6F guide and 5F diagnostic catheters), the diagnostic catheter was removed, and two guidewires were introduced into the left ventricle through the guide catheter. As a next step, one guidewire was used for a delivery sheath with a plug. (**b**) The maneuver was repeated with the second wire allowing the introduction of the second parallel delivery sheath (*arrow*). (**c**) Three AVP III plugs implanted into PVL

implanting the plug allows for easier recrossing and minimizes the risk of plug embolization. After crossing with a delivery catheter, the next plugs can be implanted as shown in Fig. 7.11b, c.

The most important part of the plug positioning and deployment is to obtain a coaxiality of the delivery sheath and the long axis of the PVL. For PVLs located close to the IAS, one of the options to improve the trajectory would be to perform the transseptal puncture through the jugular vein access. This, however, requires the particular experience of the operator. Another, simpler approach is to create the loop in the left atrium which allows for more coaxial entry into the leak channel in a manner shown in Fig. 7.12. It is usually relatively easy using the telescopic system with AL1 guide catheter (or AL2 in large atria) with 125 cm 5F JR catheter. After the puncture has been done, a 0.035–0.038″ guidewire is introduced into the atrium relatively low above the leak, forming the rail for the telescopic system. Such a system provides excellent navigation in the LA and approaching the PVL directly from above in line with the long axis of the leak. Following this, the stiff wire pre-shaped in a pigtail curve can be introduced to protect the apex and delivery sheath. It is important to maintain the loop in the atrium which can be facilitated by a gentle push on the guidewire. In a similar manner, the plugs are deployed by pulling on the delivery sheath and pushing on the wire which optimally should remain in the ventricle at this stage (requires larger sheaths). This maneuver allows to remain in line with the PVL axis.

Fig. 7.12 The delivery sheath forms a loop in the left atrium. The sheath crossed the mitral PLV located in the proximity of the intra-atrial septum

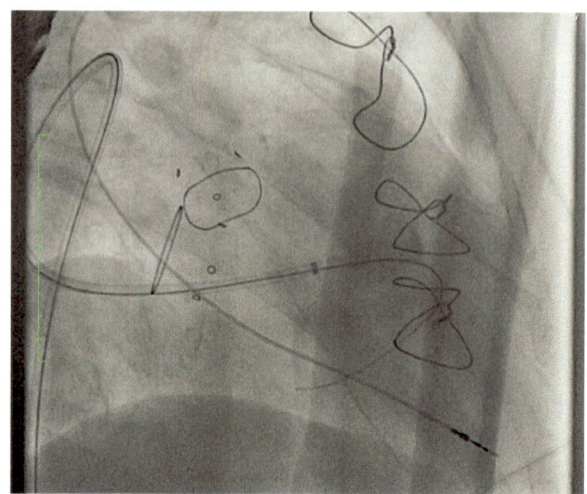

Fig. 7.13 The steerable 8.5F Agilis sheath (*arrow*) formed a telescopic system with the delivery sheath which crossed the PVL into the left ventricle

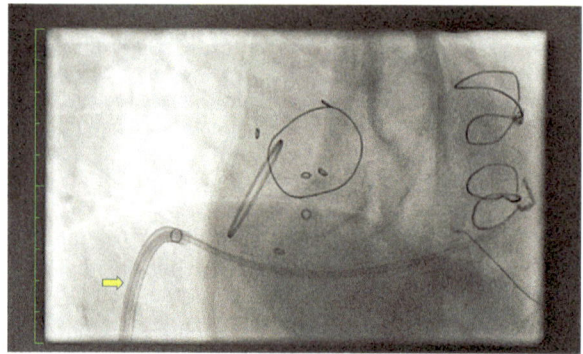

The use of steerable sheaths can facilitate procedures in PVLs located close to the septum, provided that the puncture is directly above the leak and high enough to accommodate the curvature of the steerable catheter in the LA with enough space to release the plug.

As shown in Fig. 7.13, the 8.5F Agilis sheath is used to align the delivery system with the PVL axis and introduce the guide sheath into the LV.

7.4 Leaks Located in the Proximity of LAA and Aortomitral Continuity

This localization is less challenging regarding the PVL crossing with the guidewire, but it may still lead to loss of coaxiality at the late stage of occluder deployment, especially if the softer delivery sheaths are used. The crossing can be achieved by use of the telescopic system (mother-and-child approach with 6F EBU3.5 or JR guide over a 5F long diagnostic catheter). The septal puncture site should not be too high. Usually, the middle part of the fossa ovalis is optimal.

The technical challenge as regards the delivery of the plug is shown in Fig. 7.14. An optimal approach would be to use a large (12–14F) steerable sheath to introduce a 7–8F delivery sheath/catheter as in Fig. 7.15.

If the multiplug approach is planned, either a large steerable sheath or a sequential implantation of plugs with safety wire allowing for recrossing and delivery of the second guide catheter is recommended (Fig. 7.16).

In such cases, the easiest way to proceed would be to cross the PVL with a guide catheter, introduce two exchange length guidewires, and withdraw the catheters including the access site sheath in the femoral vein. Following this, two long shuttle sheaths can be introduced over the wires. In the case of bleeding caused by two sheaths in the femoral vein, manual compression would usually be sufficient.

Fig. 7.14 PLD plug (*arrow*) implanted in mitral PVL located in the proximity of the left atrium appendage before release. The technical challenge is related to an angle between the delivery sheath and the long axis of the leak

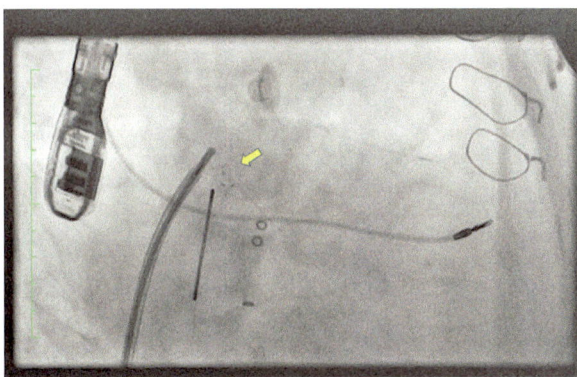

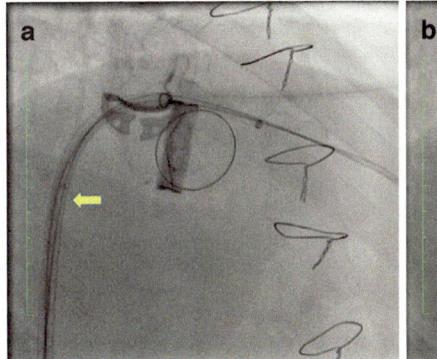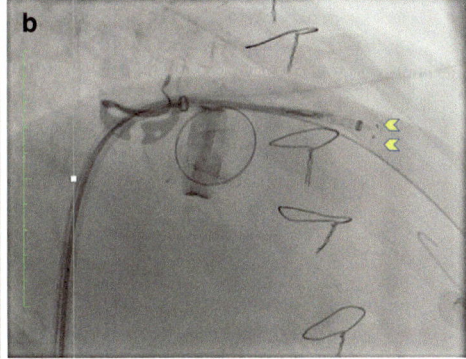

Fig. 7.15 PVL located close to aortomitral continuity. Steerable 12F FlexCath sheath used for deployment of the plugs. Panel (**a**) Steerable sheath (*arrow*) used for support of two guidewires through the PVL channel and 7F delivery sheath. Panel (**b**) Partially opened-type W rectangular PLD plug (*arrowheads*) with parallel safety wire which provides access for deployment of the second occluder. Use of large size steerable sheath allows for the enhanced rotation capability of the delivery system and facilitates the optimal orientation of the plug

Fig. 7.16 AVP III
occluders delivered
through two 7F delivery
sheaths introduced through
the single femoral vein
puncture and a single atrial
septal puncture on two
parallel wires

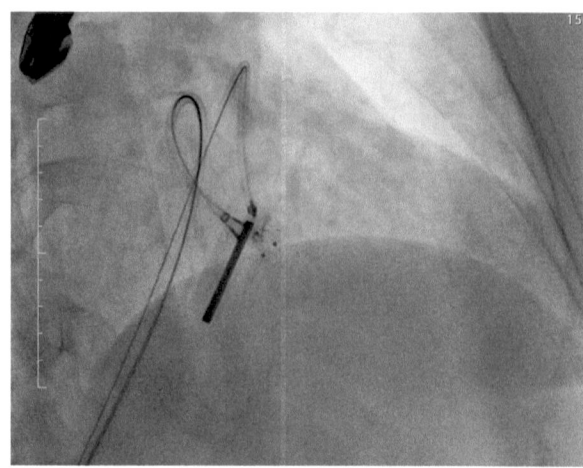

References

1. Nishimura RA, Otto CM, Bonow RO, et al. AHA/ACC guideline for the management of patients with valvular heart disease: executive summary: a report of the American College of Cardiology/American Heart Association Task Force on Practice Guidelines. J Am Coll Cardiol 2014. 2014;63:2438–88.
2. Cruz-Gonzalez I, Rama-Merchan JC, Rodriguez-Collado J, et al. Transcatheter closure of paravalvular leaks: state of the art. Neth Heart J. 2016;25:116–24.
3. Alkhouli M, Sarraf M, Maor E, et al. Techniques and outcomes of percutaneous aortic paravalvular leak closure. JACC Cardiovasc Interv. 2016;9:2416–26.
4. Giacchi G, Freixa X, Hernandez-Enriquez M, et al. Minimally invasive transradial percutaneous closure of aortic paravalvular leaks: following the steps of percutaneous coronary intervention. Can J Cardiol. 2016;32:1575 e17–9.
5. Goktekin O, Vatankulu MA, Ozhan H, et al. Early experience of percutaneous paravalvular leak closure using a novel Occlutech occluder. EuroIntervention. 2016;11:1195–200.
6. Smolka G, Pysz P, Kozlowski M, et al. Transcatheter closure of paravalvular leaks using a paravalvular leak device—a prospective Polish registry. Postepy Kardiol Interwencyjnej. 2016;12:128–34.
7. Smolka G, Pysz P, Jasinski M, et al. Multiplug paravalvular leak closure using Amplatzer Vascular Plugs III: a prospective registry. Catheter Cardiovasc Interv. 2016;87:478–87.
8. Cruz-Gonzalez I, Rama-Merchan JC, Arribas-Jimenez A, et al. Paravalvular leak closure with the Amplatzer Vascular Plug III device: immediate and short-term results. Rev Esp Cardiol (Engl Ed). 2014;67:608–14.
9. Zhou D, Pan W, Guan L, Qian J, Ge J. Retrograde transcatheter closure of mitral paravalvular leak through a mechanical aortic valve prosthesis: 2 successful cases. Tex Heart Inst J. 2016;43:137–41.

Chapter 8
Mitral Paravalvular Leak Closure: The Apical Approach

Hussam S. Suradi, Amjad Syed, Qi-Ling Cao, and Ziyad M. Hijazi

8.1 Introduction

Prosthetic paravalvular leaks (PVLs) are well-recognized complications of surgical and transcatheter valve replacement. Various series have demonstrated that 5–15% of all surgical valve replacements are complicated by some form of PVL and, specifically, 40–70% of patients who undergo transcatheter aortic valve replacement [1–3]. Significant PVL can lead to major clinical and hemodynamic consequences and impact long-term survival. Symptoms may range from a decrease in functional class to severely decompensated congestive heart failure and/or hemolysis. Furthermore, persistent PVL has been shown to increase mortality [2]. Reoperation for PVL is associated with a high recurrence rate and carries with it significant morbidity and mortality risks. With the advent of recent developments in percutaneous interventions for the treatment of structural heart disease, efforts have been made to seal PVL percutaneously by delivering occluders at the site of leak, preventing or reducing the amount of regurgitation. The percutaneous approach is now an established therapy for symptomatic patients with PVL and is frequently considered as primary therapy for eligible patients [4]. To deliver these devices, multiple

H.S. Suradi, M.D. (✉)
St Mary Medical Center, Community HealthCare Network, Hobart, IN, USA

Community Hospital, Community HealthCare Network, Munster, IN, USA

Rush Center for Structural Heart Disease, Rush University Medical Center, Chicago, IL, USA
e-mail: hussam_suradi@rush.edu

A. Syed, M.D.
St Mary Medical Center, Community HealthCare Network, Hobart, IN, USA

Community Hospital, Community HealthCare Network, Munster, IN, USA

Q.-L. Cao, M.D. • Z.M. Hijazi, M.D., M.P.H.
Sidra Cardiac Program, Sidra Medical and Research Center, Doha, Qatar

© Springer Nature Singapore Pte Ltd. 2017
G. Smolka et al. (eds.), *Transcatheter Paravalvular Leak Closure*,
DOI 10.1007/978-981-10-5400-6_8

approaches have been used, including retrograde transaortic, anterograde transseptal, and more recently transapical (TA).

TA access was first reported in 1956 by Brock et al. as a route to access the LV cavity for hemodynamic measurement [5]. Recently, the use of the TA approach has received revived interest to provide alternative access for complex cardiac structural interventions, including left ventricular pseudoaneurysm repair, ventricular septal defect closure, transcatheter aortic valve replacement, mitral valve-in-valve implantation, and, importantly, PVL closure. Two methods of the TA approach are currently utilized, open surgical (via limited thoracotomy) and completely percutaneous.

This chapter reviews the utility and technique of transcatheter mitral paravalvular leak closure using surgical and percutaneous transapical approaches.

8.2 Role of Transapical Approach in Paravalvular Leak Closure

Transapical approach provides direct access to the left ventricle for mitral and aortic PVL closure at locations that are difficult to reach via transvascular approaches (anterograde transseptal or retrograde transaortic approach) due to unfavorable angles, extensive calcifications surrounding the target lesion, or the presence of prominent papillary muscles. It can also be used as an alternative approach in patients with severe peripheral atherosclerotic disease, the presence of double mechanical valves, and for the creation of a delivery rail (transseptal-transapical, aorto-transpical) to provide additional support for the delivery system and facilitate device manipulation. The TA approach has been shown to reduce the fluoroscopic and procedural times for PVL closure in comparison to the traditional endovascular approach [6, 7]. For mitral PVLs, the TA approach provides a short and direct route to access the mitral valve. This is especially important for posteroseptal mitral PVLs, particularly those with tortuous serpiginous course, which are difficult to cross using the endovascular routes due to the steep angulations of delivery associated with these approaches.

8.3 Patient Selection

Patients who may be considered for percutaneous repair of PVL should undergo a comprehensive, multidisciplinary evaluation with close collaboration between the clinical cardiologist, interventionalist, surgeon, and imaging specialists [4]. All patients should be evaluated for active endocarditis and hemolytic anemia even in the absence of findings suspicious for these disorders, as device closure is contraindicated in active endocarditis and the presence of hemolytic anemia necessitates almost complete PVL closure. Furthermore, the surgical risk and ideal percutaneous approach for PVL closure should be discussed. The TA route should be pursued with considerable caution in patients with a hypocoagulable state due to the inherent risk of bleeding associated with the procedure. Presence of apical LV aneurysm or thrombus are absolute contraindications to TA approach. TA access should also be avoided in patients with suprasystemi pulmonary hypertension, as this group carries a significant risk of periprocedural mortality [6]. Importantly, percutaneous TA access should not be performed in patients without prior cardiac surgery, as they are considered to be at extreme risk of bleeding and tamponade because of the absence of pericardial adhesions and there is limited available data at the present time to support percutaneous TA access in the uninterrupted pericardium. TA approach should also be used with caution in senile patients as well as patients with significant left ventricular hypertrophy. In our experience the aged tissue at the apex of the heart is friable and at a risk for blow-out leading to catastrophic hemorrhage. Some operators perform a CT of the heart to assess the location of the coronary arteries and to help plan the procedure itself. Our group has not been doing this routinely. We believe that where the puncture should be done is far enough from any major coronary vessel. However, some fusion imaging technology is being used more frequently (see below).

8.4 Procedural Imaging and Guidance

8.4.1 Fluoroscopy and Echo

The role of imaging in procedural planning is an important aspect of planning for TA PVL closure and avoiding complications. In early experience, transapical access was performed without imaging, using anatomical references and pressure recordings [5, 8]. Subsequently, imaging modalities using fluoroscopy and echocardiography have been used for the guidance. Coronary angiogram prior to LV puncture can be used to define the coronary anatomy in order to avoid injury to the left anterior descending artery (LAD). Transthoracic echocardiography (TTE) can help in visualizing the LV apex and determination of the angle for puncture. In addition, TTE is helpful in evaluating for areas of myocardial wall abnormalities, exclusion of LV apical thrombus and monitoring for immediate complications such as hemopericardium. Two-dimensional, and more importantly three-dimensional transesophageal echocardiography (TEE), is used during the procedure for guiding device deployment and monitoring for complications.

8.4.2 CT and Fusion Imaging

Fluoroscopic and echocardiographic modalities are limited in demonstrating the complex three-dimensional relationship between the needle, chest wall, and left ventricle. More recently, the use of computed tomographic angiography (CTA) has been a major breakthrough in procedural planning. With 3D volume-rendered reconstruction, regional anatomy can be easily delineated. CT can provide precise distance from skin to the LV apex, help in identifying the optimal intercostal space for access and appropriate angle of needle entry into the LV as well as in identifying structures to avoid.

CT analysis and planning can be done either manually or with the use of CT-fluoroscopy fusion imaging software (HeartNavigator; Philips Healthcare, Best, The Netherlands) to guide the procedure [9]. The latter method allows the operator to fuse CT images obtained before the procedure with live fluoroscopy, improving the accuracy and safety of percutaneous transapical access. Preselected landmarks based on CT analysis are overlaid into live fluoroscopy and used for guidance of TA puncture and PVL crossing. Kliger et al. reported a series of 20 consecutive patients undergoing percutaneous LV apical access utilizing this technique. Markers were placed to identify the desired site of LV entry as well as the lung tissue and LAD artery to identify their location during LV puncture. Successful percutaneous trans-apical access was achieved in 100% of the patients, and no LV access-related complications were seen [9]. If fusion imaging software is unavailable, CTA images in equivalent angulations can be projected on a monitor adjacent to the fluoroscopic image to help guide the ventricular access [6, 10]. The latter is less reliable and heavily operator dependent. Furthermore, TEE- fluoroscopy fusion imaging software (EchoNavigator, Philips Healthcare) where TEE image is overlaid onto live fluoroscopy can be used to further guide the procedure by providing dynamic procedural guidance.

8.5   Techniques of Transapical Access

Surgical or percutaneous transapical access procedures are performed in hybrid operating rooms under general anesthesia. The patient should be prepped and draped in a sterile fashion in case emergent thoracotomy or pericardiocentesis is needed. Radiolucent defibrillator pads should be placed so as not to obscure fluoroscopic views. Two-dimensional transthoracic echocardiography (TTE) is then used to confirm that the intercostal space selected by CT analysis will provide the correct angle of entry into the lateral segment of the apex, away from the LAD artery and lung tissue. A radiopaque marker, such as a hemostat, is then placed to confirm the position and intended entry angle with fluoroscopy. To reduce the risk of lung injury, puncture should be performed at the end of expiration with the ventilator paused. After we identify the puncture site by TTE, we mark it using sterile pen, and we infiltrate it with Xylocaine. We typically use a micropuncture needle set from Cook. The needle is about 7 cm long. On occasions, with somewhat large patients, you may need to use a longer needle.

The choice of surgical or percutaneous approach to gain access into the LV cavity is governed by multiple factors, including operator preference/experience, patient characteristics, availability of imaging for procedural planning, as well as previous attempts at LV access.

8.5.1 Surgical Transapical Access

This involves a hybrid approach, with the patient under general anesthesia and the presence of both interventional and surgical teams in the hybrid operating room. A precise location of the ventricular apex is obtained using TTE guidance. Patient is positioned supine on the operating table. The left hemithorax is mildly elevated using a bump or a roll of towels extending from the inferior scapular angle to just short of anterior superior iliac spine. An anterolateral mini-thoracotomy incision measuring 4 cm is made in the skin, the appropriate intercostal space is opened, and an intercostal space retractor is then placed. The LV apex is visualized and also palpated with a finger. The apex location is now again confirmed using echo guidance.

We use an Alexis retractor which allows for a good exposure while keeping the subcutaneous fat and intercostal muscles away from the field. Two triangles of pledgeted purse-string sutures are then placed at the apex, and an access needle is introduced to puncture the apex. Once in the LV cavity, a guide wire is introduced via the needle, and the needle is exchanged for a proper sized short sheath. An appropriate activated clotting time (>250 s) using unfractionated heparin is subsequently achieved. Once PVL closure is completed, the sheath is pulled out, and the purse-string sutures are tied one after the other. Ventricle is paced at 140 beats per minute while tying the sutures to avoid tearing of the sutures. Heparin is reversed with protamine and after adequate hemostasis is obtained; a small drain is left partly in the pericardium and partly in the left pleural space to evacuate any blood that might accumulate. The intercostal space is then closed using heavy sutures and then the incision is closed in layers.

8.5.2 Percutaneous Transapical Access

If properly performed, percutaneous TA access provides a less traumatic access in comparison to surgical TA access. Once the transapical puncture site has been selected, the skin is entered with a 21-gauge micropuncture needle guided toward the site of apical entry. In most cases, the LV can be reached with a 7 cm needle, but sometimes a longer 15 cm Chiba needle (Cook, Bloomington, IN) or even 20 cm spinal needle may be needed. The needle must be introduced right on the superior border of the rib to avoid damage to the neurovascular bundle located below the inferior border of the ribs. In the absence of fusion imaging software, fluoroscopic landmarks can be used to define the location of the right ventricle (RV) (i.e., pre-existing pacer lead), the location of the left ventricle (LV gram via pigtail catheter), and the left coronary artery (selective coronary angiography). The left anterior oblique cranial view is useful when advancing the needle in the LV because it allows for visualization of all the structures mentioned, including the RV, LV, and LAD.

During puncture, contrast dye is injected through the needle to monitor the entry into the LV cavity. As mentioned above, it is helpful to hold ventilation in expiration during needle entry to prevent lung injury. After the puncture is performed, a 0.018-in.

guide wire is advanced into the left atrium or the aorta under fluoroscopic/TEE guidance. The wire is then exchanged for a micropuncture dilator, and pressure is measured to confirm position in the left ventricle prior to exchanging for a larger sheath. If the RV is inadvertently entered, the micropuncture wire or the micropuncture sheath may be removed without requiring a closure device, or it may be left in the RV temporarily as a marker during a second attempt at LV entry to avoid reentering the RV. Once position confirmed, the wire is exchanged for 0.035 in. wire through the micropuncture dilator followed by advancing an appropriately sized braided sheath. The patient is maintained at an appropriate activated clotting time (>250 s) with unfractionated heparin after the puncture.

After completing the intervention, the LV apical access may be closed with the off-label use of one of the Amplatzer closure family devices (St. Jude Medical, Inc.). Multiple devices have been used successfully to achieve closure, including the Amplatzer muscular VSD occluder, Amplatzer vascular plug II, and Amplatzer duct occluders I and II. The 6/4 mm Amplatzer duct occluder or 8 mm Amplatzer vascular plug II are the most commonly used devices. The device is introduced through the sheath, and the distal disk is opened in the LV cavity. The device is then slowly pulled back and contrast dye is injected through the side arm of the sheath to determine the location of the closure device in relationship with the LV wall. The device is pulled back until resistance is felt and the flat disk conforms to the endocardial surface. The remainder of the device is unsheathed, with the body located within the myocardium. Left ventriculography can then be performed to evaluate for any bleeding. Anticoagulation is reversed with protamine, and the subcutaneous tract is sealed with an injection of Surgiflo hemostatic matrix through the sheath while it is being removed. A final postoperative echocardiogram is performed before the patient leaves the room, to document lack of pericardial and or pleural (hemopericardium or hemothorax) effusion. Once the patient leaves the hybrid suite, we follow a strict protocol of TTE every 15 min for the first hour to look for such complications. If the echo is clear, we extend the time to every 30 min for 1 h and if that continues to be clear, we extend to every 2 h for the first 8 h. If the last echo is clear, then we perform our last echo the morning after the procedure depending on the time available in the noninvasive lab. If, at any given time, there is accumulation of fluid/blood in the pleural or pericardial space, immediate management by chest tube drainage and or pericardiocentesis should be done. From our experience, the fluid usually accumulates in the pleural space requiring chest tube.

8.6   Mitral Paravalvular Leak Closure

A 5-F steerable catheter (e.g., Angled Glidecath) is advanced through the transapical sheath, directing a 0.035 in. hydrophilic guide wire toward the mitral PVL. To cross the leak, close collaboration between the interventionalist and echocardiographer should delineate the location of the leak. Use of 3D–TEE images is crucial to show the interventionalist the location, size, and shape of the leak. The interventionalist should angulate the camera (the tube) in a view where the land marks are clear. In our lab, we believe the angulation in an LAO projection (left anterior oblique about 40° with some cranial angulation about 15–20°) will help the interventionalist determine where to place the angled catheter (JR or angled Glidecath). After the leak is crossed with the wire and the position confirmed by 3D–TEE and fluoroscopy, the catheter is advanced across the defect into the left atrium. We check LA pressure here after removing the wire. Then an extra-support, exchange-length wire is placed. The catheter is then exchanged for an appropriately sized sheath or guide catheter, depending on the device to be used. Difficulty advancing the catheter and/or sheath may require the creation of an exteriorized arteriovenous delivery rail (transapical and transseptal) to provide additional support for the delivery system and facilitate device manipulation. After the sheath is across the PVL, the closure device is passed through the sheath. In the USA, there are no devices that are designed specifically for PVL closure approved; therefore, the Amplatzer family of occluders is the most commonly used devices in an off-label fashion (Fig. 8.1). The distal disk is opened in the left atrium and pulled back slowly until resistance is felt, followed by deployment of the proximal disk in the ventricular side. For large PVLs, multiple devices might need to be deployed either sequentially or simultaneously. The closure device is then released if an appropriate reduction in regurgitation is seen on TEE without prosthetic valve interference. Outside the USA, there are devices designed specifically for closure of paravalvular mitral leaks (Fig. 8.1): Occlutech PLD devices and Amplatzer vascular plug III [11–14].

8.7   Outcomes

Complications can be divided into those related to TA access and PVL closure. Potential transapical access complications include hemothorax, pericardial effusion, coronary laceration, LV pseudoaneurysm, pneumothorax, cardiac arrhythmia, and death. Hemothorax is the most frequent complication and can be related to coronary or intercostal vessel laceration or bleeding from the LV puncture site. Potential complications related to PVL closure include prosthetic valve interference by device, device embolization, stroke, increased hemolysis, vascular complications, and death.

Good technical success has been reported with both surgical [15, 16] and percutaneous TA PVL closure [6, 17]. In the largest series by Jelnin et al., 28 patients underwent 32 percutaneous transapical punctures. Complications were observed in two patients (7.1%). The complications encountered included pericardial effusion and death. The death occurred in a patient with suprasystemic pulmonary hypertension resulting in electromechanical dissociation following LV apical access [6]. The literature related to TA PVL closure is still limited and more experience is still needed to improve the technical steps and outcome of this procedure.

In a case we recently have done, a patient presented with severe paravalvular mitral leak resulting in severe heart failure and moderate hemolysis. She was taken

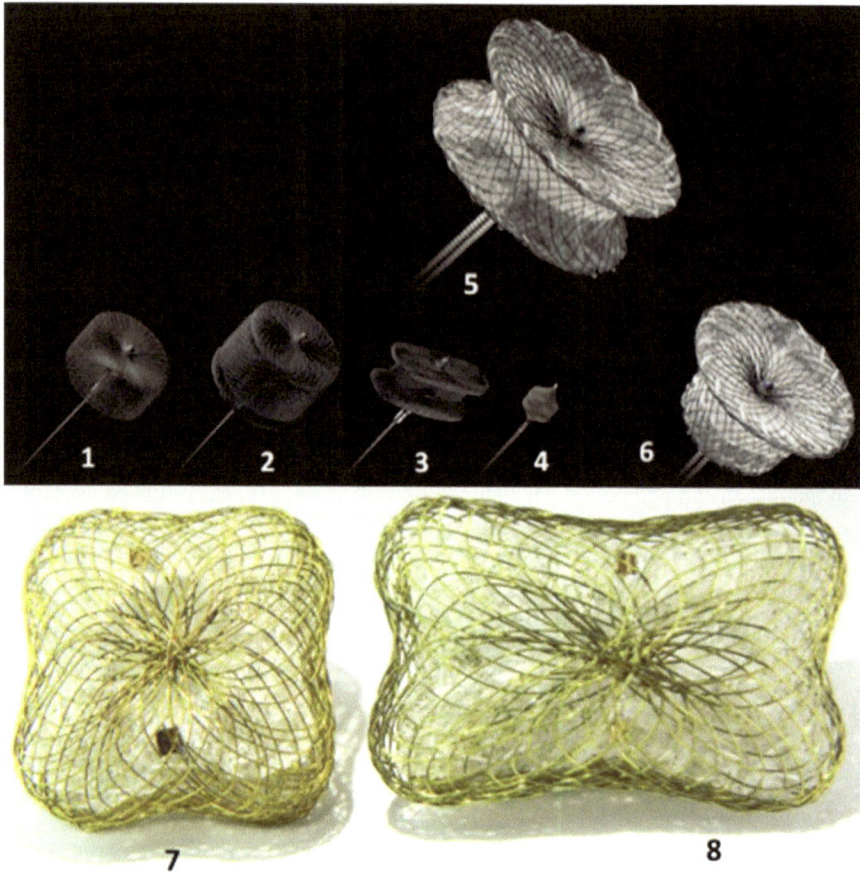

Fig. 8.1 The Amplatzer family of devices (*1*, Amplatzer vascular plug I; *2*, vascular plug II; *3*, vascular plug III; *4*, vascular plug IV; *5*, muscular VSD device; *6*, Amplatzer Duct Occluder) and Occlutech PLD devices; *7*, square device; *8*, rectangular device)

to the hybrid suite and underwent mitral PVL closure via the percutaneous transapical approach. She had two large leaks in the posteromedial aspect of the mitral valve ring. Prior to closure, her LA pressure was remarkable for an "a" wave of 33 mmHg, "v" wave of 70 mmHg, and mean pressure of 32 mmHg. The first device we used was a 10 mm × 5 mm Occlutech rectangular device. However there was a residual leak, and, unfortunately, we did not have at that time another large rectangular device, and, therefore, a 10 mm Amplatzer muscular VSD device was used. The majority of leak has disappeared, and there was a small residual leak between the devices. We thought this should get better over time. However, that same day, she started to experience significant hemolysis requiring transfusions on a daily basis, and, finally, after 1 week of no improvement in the hemolysis, we decided to take her back to the hybrid suite to close the residual leak. Of note, her heart failure symptoms had improved significantly.

We accessed her LV percutaneously from the apex using a different puncture site in the apex, and we identified the residual leak to be between the devices. After crossing this leak, LA pressure showed significant improvement ("a" wave was 23 mmHg, "v" wave 50 mmHg, and mean 23 mmHg). To eliminate the entire leak without leaving chance for residual leak, we used a 25 mm Amplatzer cribriform device (St. Jude Medical, Inc.). The device after deployment eliminated the residual leak completely and was close to the mitral valve leaflets without causing significant obstruction (mean mitral inflow gradient was about 5–6 mmHg). The procedure was successful to the extent that, at the end of the procedure, the urine color started to clear up in the Foley's catheter (Fig. 8.2). Figures 8.3 and 8.4 demonstrate the fluoroscopic and echocardiographic images of the first and second procedures to close the paravalvular leaks.

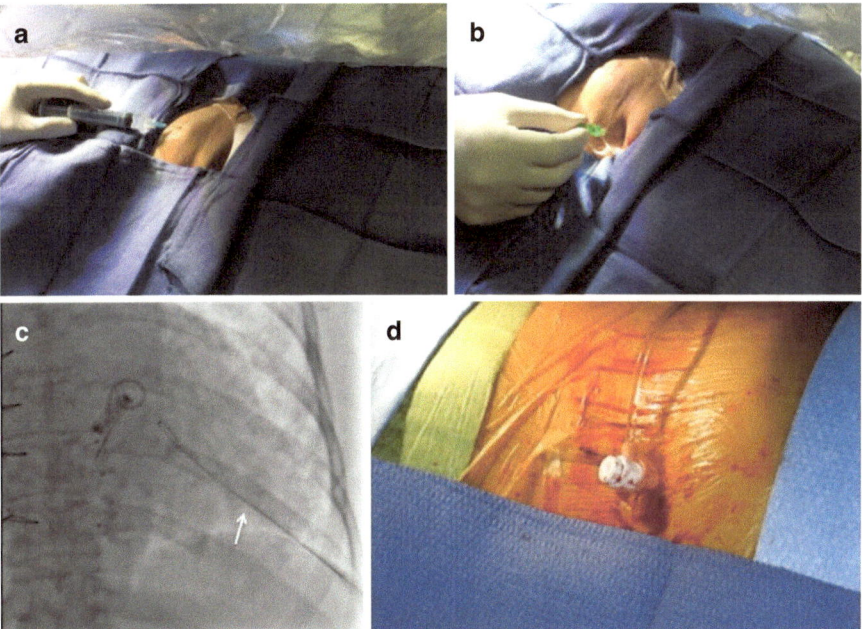

Fig. 8.2 Foley's catheter during second procedure, after deployment of the last device. Urine before closure shows the hemolysis (*red arrow*) and fresh urine is clear (*white arrow*)

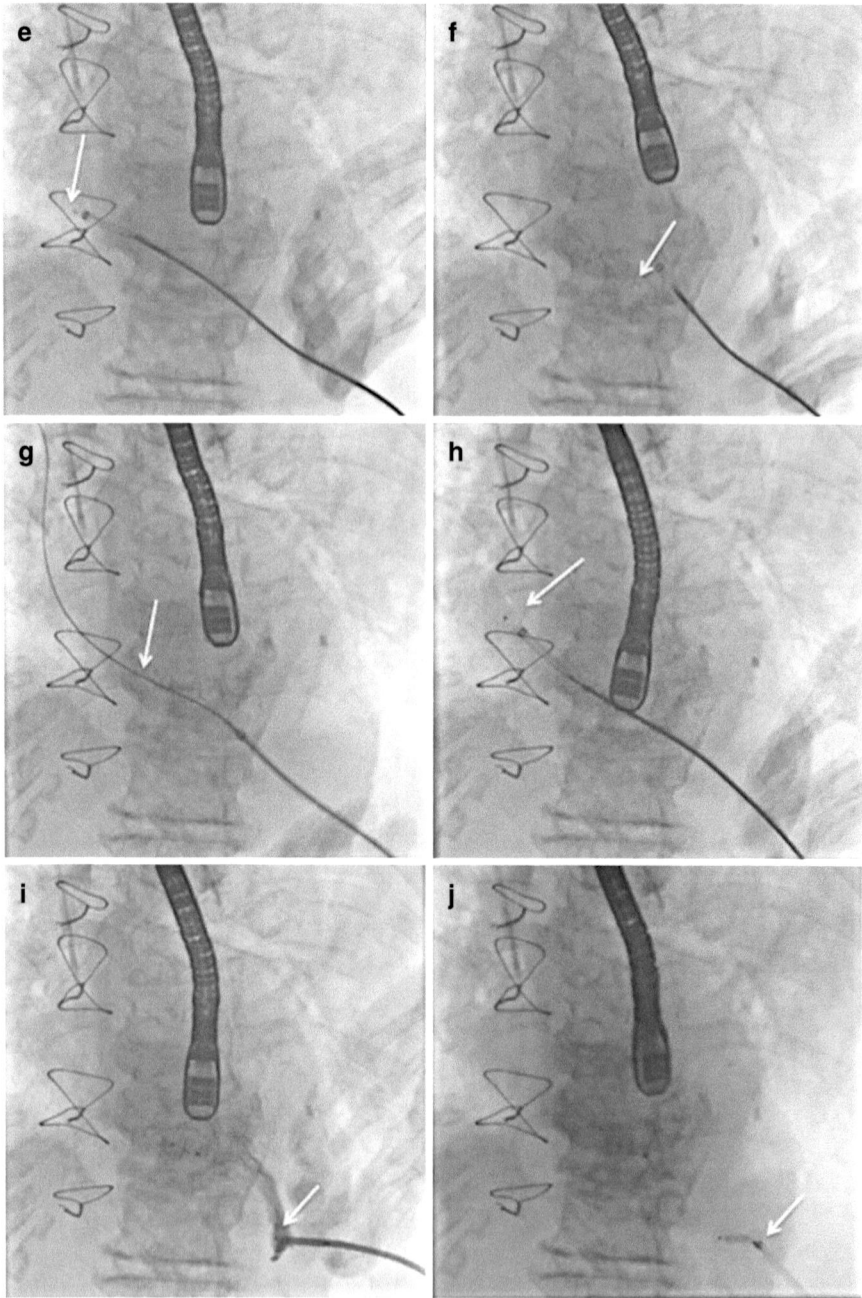

Fig. 8.2 (continued)

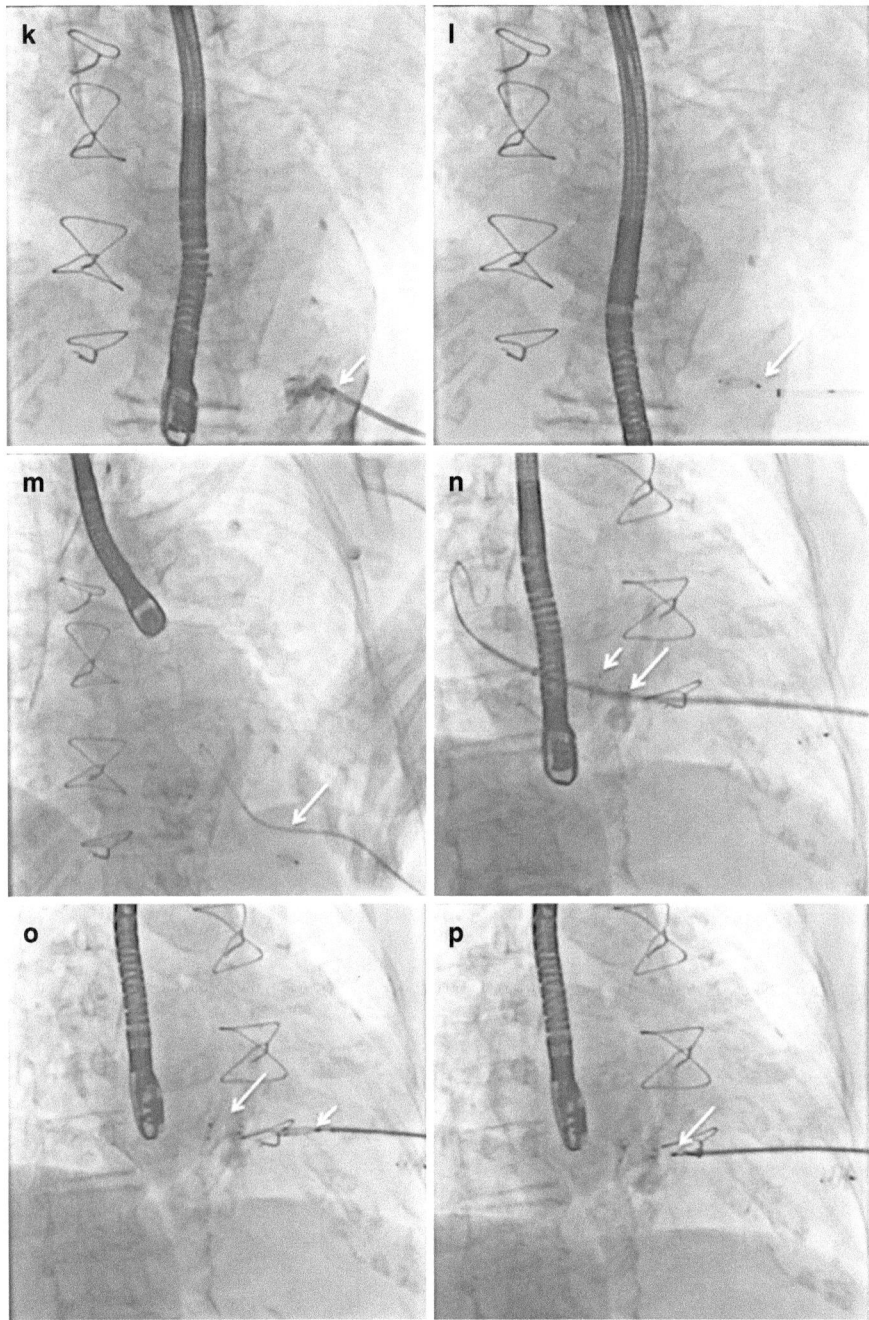

Fig. 8.2 (continued)

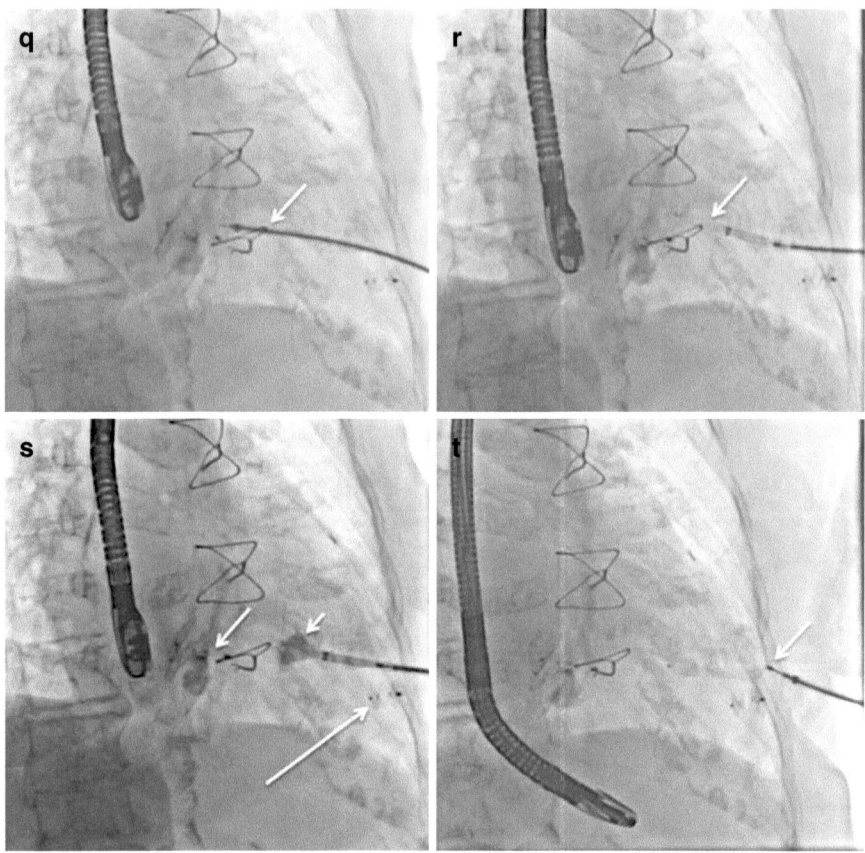

Fig. 8.2 (continued)

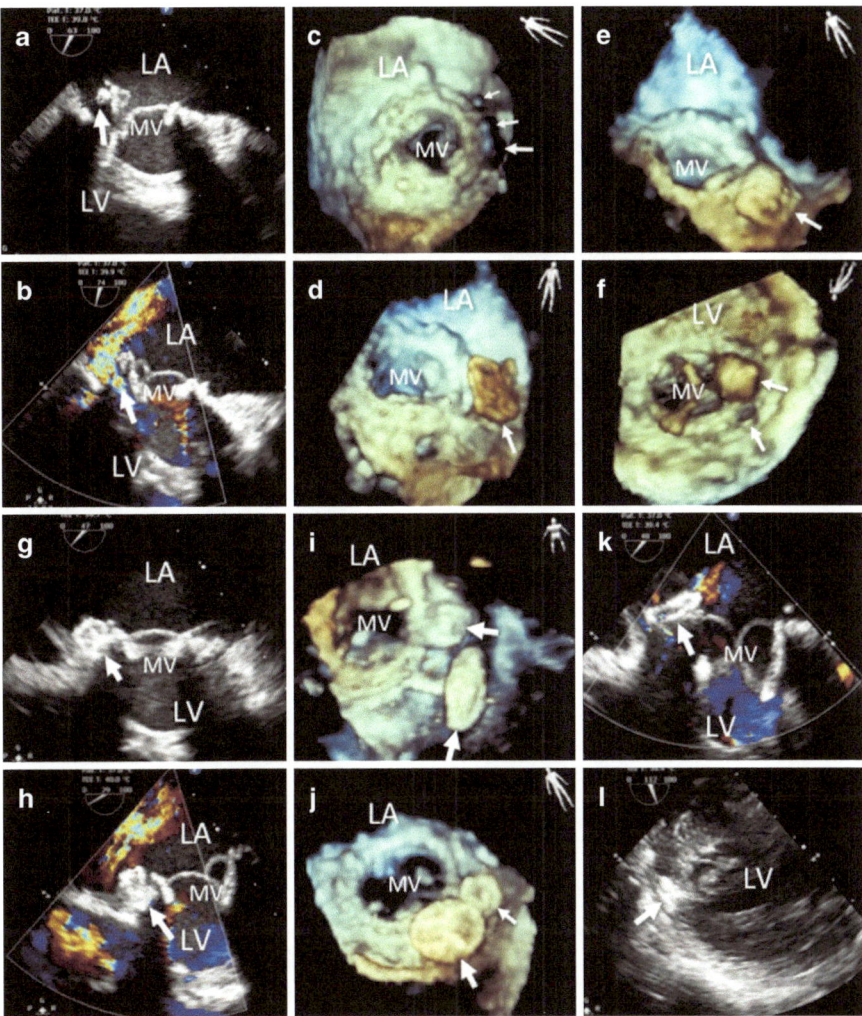

Fig. 8.3 The steps of percutaneous TA access in an 84-year-old female patient status post bioprosthetic mitral valve replacement. (**a**) Infiltration of the skin with Xylocaine. (**b**) Use of micropuncture needle (0.021 in. gauge) to puncture the LV percutaneously. (**c**) Passage of the wire (*arrow*) into the left ventricle cavity. (**d**) Over the wire, a 7-Fr sheath was inserted and positioned in the LV cavity. (**e**) A delivery sheath with the Occlutech rectangular device (*arrow*) at the tip of the sheath. (**f**) The device (*arrow*) has been released at its location. (**g**) Passage of a wire (*arrow*) in the residual defect beside the already released device. (**h**) Deployment of one desk (*arrow*) of a muscular VSD device in the left atrial side of the defect. (**i**) Closure of the track with a vascular plug II (*arrow*). One desk is in the endocardium of the left ventricle. (**j**) Pulling the proximal desk of the plug into the epicardium (*arrow*). (**k**) Angiogram via side arm of the short sheath to confirm position of the plug (*arrow*). (**l**) Release of the plug (*arrow*). (**m**) Puncture of the left ventricle apex for the second procedure beside the first puncture site (*arrow*). (**n**) Passage of a sheath beside the first two devices (*short-arrow* VSD device; *long-arrow* Occlutech device). (**o**) Deployment of the left atrial desk (*arrow*) of a 25 mm cribriform device. (**p**) Deployment of the ventricular desk of the device while still attached (*arrow*). (**q**) Release of the device (*arrow*). (**r**) Deployment of muscular VSD device to close the track (*arrow*). (**s**) Angiogram via side arm of the sheath to position the VSD device (*short arrow*), medium size arrow shows last device deployed in the defect and long arrow shows the old vascular plug II used to close the track in the first procedure. (**t**) The muscular VSD device was positioned in the correct position (one part in the epicardium)

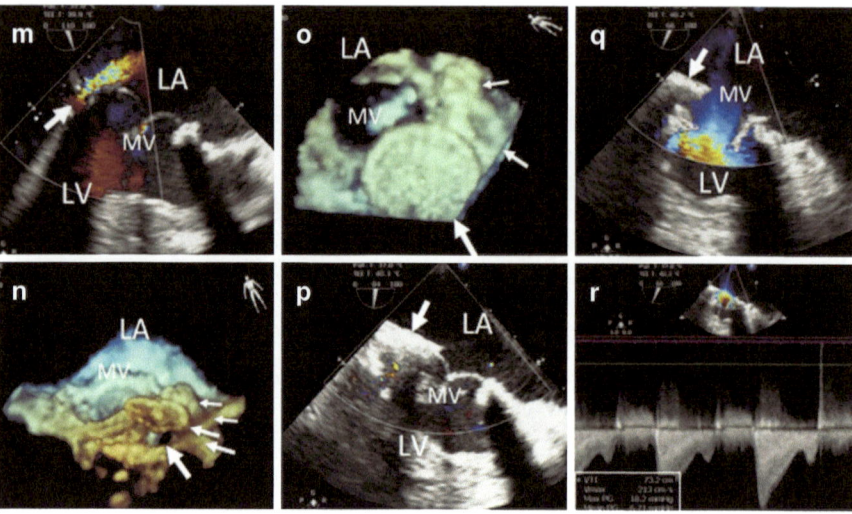

Fig. 8.3 (continued)

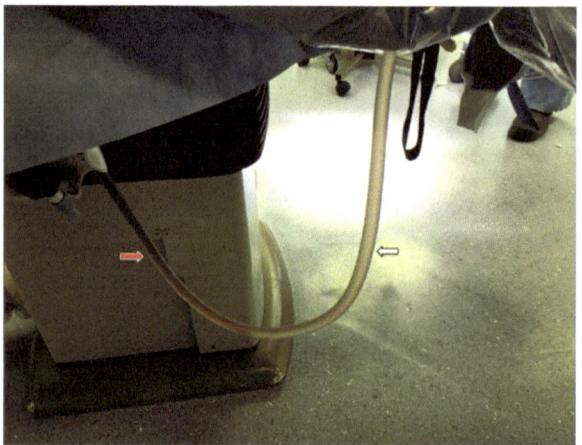

Fig. 8.4 Transesophageal echocardiographic images (2D and 3D) of the closure procedure. (**a, b**) Two-chamber view without and with color Doppler showing the leak (*arrow*). *LA* left atrium, *LV* left ventricle. (**c**) 3D–TEE image from LA showing large leak (*arrows*). (**d**) Same view as c, showing the 10 × 5 mm Occlutech PLD device (*arrow*) deployed in the left atrium. (**e, f**) Same view as **c** showing the device released (*arrow*) in the anterior part of the defect and the other arrow shows residual leak posterior. (**g, h**) 2D–TEE images without and with color Doppler showing device in position (*arrow*) and residual leak. (**i, j**) 3D images from left atrium showing the second device (*arrow*) being positioned in the residual leak. *Small arrow* indicates first device. (**k**) 2D image showing the device (*arrow*) in good position with small residual leak. (**l**) image showing the vascular plug II positioned in the endocardium (*arrow*) to close the track. (**m**) 2D image with color Doppler showing the residual leak (*arrow*). (**n**) 3D image showing the first two devices (*small arrows*) and the residual leak (*large arrow*). (**o-p**) The left atrial desk of the 25 mm cribriform device opened in the left atrium (*large arrow*). *Small arrows* are the first two devices. (**q**) After the device has been released (*arrow*) showing no residual leak at all. (**r**) Doppler across the mitral valve showing mild mitral valve stenosis with mean gradient of 6 mmHg

8.8 Summary

Transapical access for PVL is a safe approach with a low rate of access-site complications. It carries the advantage of providing a short pathway between the apex and mitral valve, facilitating closure for anatomically difficult PVLs, such as those with calcified tortuous tracts and posteroseptal (medial) mitral PVLs, decreasing both fluoroscopy and procedural times. Careful procedural planning utilizing multimodality imaging is essential to avoid complications, providing more accurate and safer means of access. Equally important to LV entry is transapical closure. Amplatzer devices have been used for apical closure with good results; however, long-term follow-up data is still needed. The development of percutaneous apical closure devices {e.g., CardiApex (Cardiapex Ltd., Or Akiva, Israel) and Safex (Comed, Bolsward, Netherlands) devices} specifically designed to work in a closed-chest transapical setting represents an important step toward further development of the transapical percutaneous technique, as it will further simplify and standardize the transapical transcatheter technique [18]. Further, we should stress on the importance of closing the entire leak and to avoid leaving behind any residual jets as, on occasion, these may result in more hemolysis secondary to flow turbulence leading to excessive shearing forces on the red blood cells.

References

1. Davila-Roman VG, Waggoner AD, Kennard ED, Holubkov R, Jamieson WR, Englberger L, et al. Prevalence and severity of paravalvular regurgitation in the artificial valve endocarditis reduction trial (AVERT) echocardiography study. J Am Coll Cardiol. 2004;44(7):1467–72. Epub 2004/10/07.
2. Kodali SK, Williams MR, Smith CR, Svensson LG, Webb JG, Makkar RR, et al. Two-year outcomes after transcatheter or surgical aortic-valve replacement. N Engl J Med. 2012;366(18):1686–95. Epub 2012/03/27.
3. Hahn RT, Pibarot P, Stewart WJ, Weissman NJ, Gopalakrishnan D, Keane MG, et al. Comparison of transcatheter and surgical aortic valve replacement in severe aortic stenosis: a longitudinal study of echocardiography parameters in cohort a of the PARTNER trial (placement of aortic transcatheter valves). J Am Coll Cardiol. 2013;61(25):2514–21. Epub 2013/04/30.
4. Nishimura RA, Otto CM, Bonow RO, Carabello BA, Erwin JP III, Guyton RA, et al. 2014 AHA/ACC guideline for the management of patients with valvular heart disease: a report of the American College of Cardiology/American Heart Association task force on practice guidelines. J Thorac Cardiovasc Surg. 2014;148(1):e1–e132. Epub 2014/06/19.
5. Brock R, Milstein BB, Ross DN. Percutaneous left ventricular puncture in the assessment of aortic stenosis. Thorax. 1956;11(3):163–71. Epub 1956/09/01.
6. Jelnin V, Dudiy Y, Einhorn BN, Kronzon I, Cohen HA, Ruiz CE. Clinical experience with percutaneous left ventricular transapical access for interventions in structural heart defects a safe access and secure exit. JACC Cardiovasc Interv. 2011;4(8):868–74. Epub 2011/08/20.
7. Ruiz CE, Jelnin V, Kronzon I, Dudiy Y, Del Valle-Fernandez R, Einhorn BN, et al. Clinical outcomes in patients undergoing percutaneous closure of periprosthetic paravalvular leaks. J Am Coll Cardiol. 2011;58(21):2210–7. Epub 2011/11/15.

8. Levy MJ, Lillehei CW. Percutaneous direct cardiac Catheterization. A new method, with results in 122 patients. N Engl J Med. 1964;271:273–80. Epub 1964/08/01.

9. Kliger C, Jelnin V, Sharma S, Panagopoulos G, Einhorn BN, Kumar R, et al. CT angiography-fluoroscopy fusion imaging for percutaneous transapical access. JACC Cardiovasc Imaging. 2014;7(2):169–77. Epub 2014/01/15.

10. Davidavicius G, Rucinskas K, Drasutiene A, Samalavicius R, Bilkis V, Zakarkaite D, et al. Hybrid approach for transcatheter paravalvular leak closure of mitral prosthesis in high-risk patients through transapical access. J Thorac Cardiovasc Surg. 2014;148(5):1965–9. Epub 2014/06/04.

11. Goktekin O, Vatankulu MA, Tasal A, Sonmez O, Basel H, Topuz U, et al. Transcatheter trans-apical closure of paravalvular mitral and aortic leaks using a new device: first in man experience. Catheter Cardiovasc Interv. 2014;83(2):308–14. Epub 2013/05/25.

12. Goktekin O, Vatankulu MA, Ozhan H, Ay Y, Ergelen M, Tasal A, et al. Early experience of percutaneous paravalvular leak closure using a novel Occlutech occluder. EuroIntervention. 2016;11(10):1195–200. Epub 2016/02/22.

13. Smolka G, Pysz P, Jasinski M, Roleder T, Peszek-Przybyla E, Ochala A, et al. Multiplug paravalvular leak closure using Amplatzer vascular plugs III: a prospective registry. Catheter Cardiovasc Interv. 2016;87(3):478–87. Epub 2015/05/13.

14. Cruz-Gonzalez I, Rama-Merchan JC, Arribas-Jimenez A, Rodriguez-Collado J, Martin-Moreiras J, Cascon-Bueno M, et al. Paravalvular leak closure with the Amplatzer vascular plug III device: immediate and short-term results. Rev Esp Cardiol (Engl Ed). 2014;67(8):608–14. Epub 2014/07/20.

15. Swaans MJ, Post MC, van der Ven HA, Heijmen RH, Budts W, ten Berg JM. Transapical treatment of paravalvular leaks in patients with a logistic EuroSCORE of more than 15%: acute and 3-month outcomes of a "proof of concept" study. Catheter Cardiovasc Interv. 2012;79(5):741–7. Epub 2011/08/02.

16. Brown SC, Boshoff DE, Rega F, Eyskens B, Budts W, Heidbuchel H, et al. Transapical left ventricular access for difficult to reach interventional targets in the left heart. Catheter Cardiovasc Interv. 2009;74(1):137–42. Epub 2009/05/01.

17. Sorajja P, Cabalka AK, Hagler DJ, Rihal CS. Percutaneous repair of paravalvular prosthetic regurgitation: acute and 30-day outcomes in 115 patients. Circ Cardiovasc Interv. 2011;4(4):314–21. Epub 2011/07/28.

18. Ferrari E. Apical access and closure devices for transapical transcatheter heart valve procedures. Swiss Med Wkly. 2016;146:w14237. Epub 2016/02/24.

Chapter 9
Paravalvular Leakage After Transcatheter Aortic Valve Implantation

Zouhair Rahhab and Nicolas M. Van Mieghem

9.1 Introduction

Transcatheter aortic valve implantation (TAVI) is the treatment of choice for inoperable or high-risk patients with severe aortic stenosis and is now expanding to intermediate- and low-risk patients [1–3]. A frequently seen complication after TAVI is paravalvular leakage (PVL), which is considered the Achilles' heel of TAVI since several studies have shown an association with worse outcome [4–6]. Several trials and registries reported PVL rates ranging from 40% to 67% for trivial-mild leaks and from 7% to 20% for moderate-severe leaks [1, 7]. The wide variability of these frequencies may be partly related to the transcatheter heart valve (THV) design but may also reflect different methodologies for PVL assessment. Accurate PVL quantification remains challenging since there is no standardized method yet.

It is important to understand the underlying mechanisms in order to prevent/minimize and treat PVL. In recent years the PVL incidence may have declined because of growing experience, improved implantation techniques, and the incorporation of sealing fabric around the valve frame with newer-generation THVs.

Z. Rahhab, M.D.
Department of Cardiology, Thoraxcenter, Erasmus Medical Center, Rotterdam, The Netherlands

N.M. Van Mieghem, M.D., Ph.D. (✉)
Department of Interventional Cardiology, Thoraxcenter, ErasmusMC, Room Bd 171 's Gravendijkwal 230, 3015 CE Rotterdam, The Netherlands
e-mail: n.vanmieghem@erasmusmc.nl

© Springer Nature Singapore Pte Ltd. 2017
G. Smolka et al. (eds.), *Transcatheter Paravalvular Leak Closure*,
DOI 10.1007/978-981-10-5400-6_9

9.2 Assessment of PVL

9.2.1 Angiographic Assessment

Contrast angiography can be used for semiquantitative assessment of aortic regurgitation (AR). AR severity is visually assessed according to the Sellers classification [8] which is based on the density of left ventricular opacification: Grade 1 (mild) corresponds with a small amount of contrast entering the left ventricle (LV) in diastole without filling the entire cavity and clearing with each cardiac cycle; Grade 2 (moderate) corresponds with contrast filling of the entire LV in diastole with faint opacification of the entire LV; Grade 3 (moderate to severe) corresponds with contrast filling and opacification of the entire LV in diastole, equal in density to the ascending aorta; Grade 4 (severe) corresponds with contrast filling of the entire LV in diastole on the first beat with denser opacification than the ascending aorta.

9.2.1.1 Limitations

AR interpretation by aortography is subjective and has high interobserver variability. Several technical factors (e.g., position of the pigtail catheter and contrast volume/injection rate) may contribute to this variability. Furthermore, aortography weighs the total amount of contrast leaking into the LV ventricle and cannot distinguish between trans- and paravalvular leakage. In addition, iodinated contrast is needed which increases the risk of acute kidney injury (AKI).

9.2.2 Video Densitometry

Dedicated software for semiautomated AR quantification may improve inter- and intra-observer variability of contrast aortography. The principle relies on time-dependent changes in contrast distribution and density within the LV during diastole [9]. The software produces five time-density curves (aortic root (reference area), left ventricular base, mid, apex, and overall) and measures the relative area under the curve to obtain the quantified aortic regurgitation index (qAR index) with values ranging from 0.0 (no AR) to 4.0 (severe AR).

Suboptimal contrast angiography studies including incomplete visualization of the LV apex and superposition of the spine and the abdominal aorta may affect its feasibility and accuracy. To address these issues, a simplified video densitometric analysis restricted to the LVOT (LVOT-AR) has been proposed with acceptable results. A recent study showed that LVOT-AR was feasible in 64.8% of aortograms vs. 29.7% for qAR index. Interobserver variability for LVOT-AR was low (mean difference ± standard deviation; 0.01 ± 0.05, $p = 0.53$), and interobserver correlation was high ($r = 0.95$, $p < 0.001$) [10].

9.2.3 Hemodynamic Assessment

The aortic regurgitation index (AR index) relies on the difference between the invasively measured diastolic central blood pressure (DBP) and the left ventricle end-diastolic pressure (LVEDP) divided by the systolic blood pressure (SBP) × 100 [(DBP − LVEDP/SBP] × 100) (Fig. 9.1 and 9.2) [11]. The seminal paper on this topic illustrated that AR index decreases in parallel with increasing severity of PVL, from 31.7 ± 10.4 in patients without PVL to 28.0 ± 8.5 in patients with mild PVL, 19.6 ± 7.6 in patients with moderate PVL, and 7.6 ± 2.6 in patients with severe PVL ($p < 0.001$). AR index <25 was an independent predictor for 1-year mortality (hazard ratio 2.9, 95% confidence interval 1.3–6.4; $p = 0.009$) [11]. Elevation of the LVEDP due to volume loading, diastolic dysfunction, or periprocedural myocardial ischemia can result in a lower diastolic transvalvular gradient and thus a "false-positive" AR index [11]. Diastolic hemodynamic parameters can be influenced by heart rate [12], and this is not taken into account in the AR index. Finally, the AR index does not differentiate between transvalvular and paravalvular leakage.

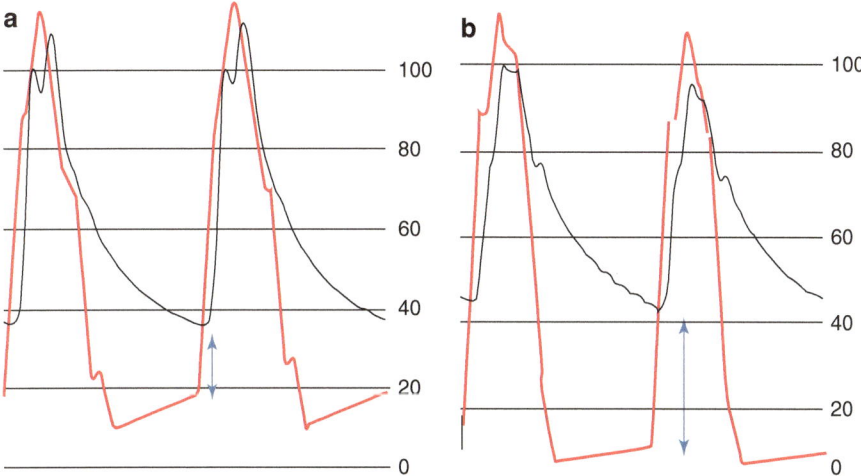

Fig. 9.1 Hemodynamic assessment of a patient (**a**) with and (**b**) without PVL. (**a**) AR index patient A = (37 − 18)/111 × 100 = 17. (**b**) AR index patient B = (42 − 10)/105 × 100 = 30

Index	Definition	Cut-off	PVL > mild Specificity	1-year mortality Specificity
AR-index (ARI)	$\dfrac{\text{Diastolic blood pressure} - \text{Left ventricle end diastolic pressure} \times 100}{\text{Systolic blood pressure}}$	<25	75.1%	75%
ARI ratio in addition to ARI post	$\dfrac{\text{ARI post ; ARI post}}{\text{ARI pre}}$	<0.60; <25	93.2%	93.3%
Diastolic pressure time index$_{adj}$	$\dfrac{\text{Diastolic pressure time index} \times 100}{\text{Systolic blood pressure}}$	< 27.9	N.A.	N.A.

Fig. 9.2 Overview of different hemodynamic indices with their definition, cutoff values, and specificity. *N.A.* not available

ARI ratio correlates ARI before and after transcatheter valve implantation. The ARI ratio with a cutoff <0.60 improved the specificity for the prediction of more than mild PVL and 1-year mortality from 75.1% to 93.2% and from 75.0% to 93.3%, respectively (Fig. 9.2) [13].

The diastolic pressure-time (DPT) index is calculated by measuring the area between the aortic and left ventricular pressure-time curves during diastole and divided by the duration of diastole. DPT index is adjusted for the SBP (DPT index-$_{adj}$ = (DPT index/SBP) × 100) [14].

DPT index$_{adj}$ decreases with significant PVL (grade ≥ 2), and a value ≤ 27.9 seems associated with 1-year mortality (hazard ratio 2.5, 95% confidence interval; 1.3–6.4); $p < 0.001$ (Fig. 9.2) [14].

9.2.4 Echocardiographic Assessment

The Valve Academic Research Consortium-2 (VARC-2) recommends Doppler echocardiography for the quantitative and semiquantitative assessment of PVL [15]. Color Doppler echocardiography can distinguish between trans- and paravalvular leakage; for the evaluation of PVL, Color Doppler should be performed just below the valve stent, whereas for the evaluation of transvalvular leakage, it should be performed at the coaptation point of the leaflets [15]. All imaging windows should be assessed in order to ensure complete visualization of PVL; however the parasternal short-axis view is critical in assessing the number and severity of paravalvular jets [15].

Transesophageal echocardiography (TEE) may improve PVL assessment in patients in whom poor images are obtained by transthoracic echocardiography (TTE); however TEE is more invasive.

Current trends to perform TAVI under local anesthesia or (mild) conscious sedation limit TEE feasibility. Furthermore TTE assessment in the cath lab is challenging because the patient is in the supine position (no left lateral decubitus). In addition, TTE may mask PVL jets located posteriorly, whereas TEE may mask jets located anteriorly.

9.2.4.1 Limitations

Most echocardiographic parameters (Fig. 9.3) used for the assessment of PVL are based on surgical heart valves and are not validated in transcatheter heart valves. In addition, several studies suggest that echocardiography underestimates the severity of PVL when compared to cardiac magnetic resonance (CMR) [16, 17].

Recently, Geleijnse et al. showed that the parasternal short-axis analysis of the circumferential extent of PVL, which is recommended by the VARC-2 and is considered critical in assessing PVL, was false negative in 14% of cases. This may imply underestimation of PVL in prior studies relying on circumferential PVL extent [18].

		Prosthetic aortic valve regurgitation	
	Mild	Moderate	Severe
Semiquantitave parameters			
Diastolic flow reversal in the descending aorta - PW	Absent or brief early diastolic	Intermediate	Prominent holodiastolic
Circumferential extent of prosthetic valve paravalvular regurgitation (%)	< 10%	10% – 29%	≥ 30%
Quantitative parameters			
Regurgitation volume (mL./beat)	< 30 mL	30 –59 mL	≥ 60 mL
Regurgitation fraction (%)	< 30%	30% – 49%	≥ 50%
EROA (cm²)	0.10 cm²	0.10 – 0.29 cm²	≥ 0.30 cm²

Fig. 9.3 VARC-2 echocardiography criteria for the quantification of PVL adapted from Kappetein et al. *PW* pulsed wave, *EROA* effective regurgitation orifice area

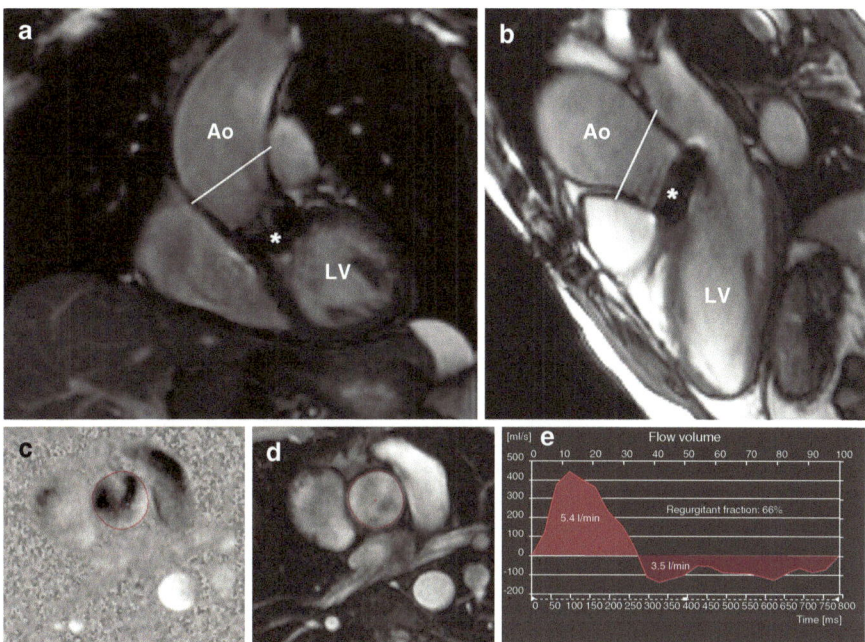

Fig. 9.4 Example of aortic regurgitation quantification with cardiac magnetic resonance (CMR) by using phase-contrast velocity technique. (**a** and **b**) Coronal and three-chamber views (*white line* represents the level of flow measurement and *asterisk* (*) the valve in aortic position), (**c** and **d**) Phase-contrast velocity and anatomic images, (**e**) Graphic of flow measurement showing a regurgitation fraction of 66%. Image courtesy of Raluca Chelu, MD, Department of Radiology, Erasmus Medical Center

9.2.5   Cardiac Magnetic Resonance (CMR)

Cardiac magnetic resonance is a noninvasive imaging modality allowing accurate and reproducible quantification of aortic regurgitation (AR) by using phase-contrast velocity mapping technique [16, 17]. A phase-contrast view in a short-axis plane just above the THV is obtained for quantification of the forward and reversed flow volumes (Fig. 9.4) [16]. The regurgitation fraction (RF), which is defined as the diastolic reversed flow volume/systolic forward volume × 100, can be used as a parameter for the stratification of the severity of PVL. None/trivial corresponds with a RF of <8%; mild corresponds with a RF of 9–20%; moderate corresponds with a RF of 21–39%; severe corresponds with a RF of >40% [16, 17].

9.2.5.1 Limitations

Since CMR is not available in the catheterization room, intra-procedural assessment of PVL is not possible and thereby not contributing in the decision-making whether to perform additional corrective maneuvers. In addition, CMR does not differentiate between transvalvular and paravalvular leakage. The cutoff values of the RF, used for the stratification of PVL, are not validated.

Also, TAVI-induced conduction abnormalities may require a permanent pacemaker or implantable cardioverter defibrillator (ICD) which is at least a relative contraindication for CMR (even for the MR-compatible devices).

9.2.6 Biomarkers

Recently van Belle et al. demonstrated that changes in von Willebrand factor during TAVI can predict the presence of PVL [19]. Defects in von Willebrand factor high-molecular-weight (HMW) multimers occur in patients with PVL, through turbulent blood flow caused by paravalvular leakage. The HMW multimer conformation changes lead to proteolytic cleavage [19]. This may shorten HMW multimers that are less hemostatically competent and cause a prolongation of the closure time with adenosine diphosphate (CT-ADP).

CT-ADP decreased in patients with no regurgitation post-TAVI from 235 ± 62 (baseline) to 129 ± 54 s (end of procedure), while in patients with persistent AR, CT-ADP remained high throughout the procedure. In the corrected regurgitation group (i.e., post-balloon dilatation or second valve), the CT-ADP did not change markedly from 250 ± 53 (baseline) to 223 ± 49 s (after valve implantation) but decreased after the corrective procedure to 124 ± 59 s. These findings were also confirmed in a validation cohort: The CT-ADP at the end of the procedure was significantly higher in patients with aortic regurgitation than in those without regurgitation (244 ± 64 s vs. 118 ± 53 s, $p < 0.001$ [19].

9.3 Determinants of PVL

9.3.1 Patient-Related Factors

– Native Aortic Valve Calcification
  In contrast to surgical aortic valve replacement, the calcified native aortic valve is not excised with TAVI. In fact, valvular calcification is needed to ensure anchoring of the THV. We previously demonstrated that patients with valve dislodgement had

significantly less aortic root calcification (Agatston score median 1951 AU (IQR, 799–3103) vs. 3289 AU (IQR 2097–4481), $p = 0.016$) with an Agatston score <2359 AU as a single independent predictor for valve dislodgement (OR 3.10, 1.09–8.84 [20]. However, excessive calcification of the aortic annulus (Fig. 9.5) might lead to frame under expansion and incomplete circumferential apposition (of the THV) to the native annulus [21–23]. Amount and distribution of annular calcification are a predictor for PVL [24–27]. A study on [27] 112 consecutively treated patients confirmed a significant association between the aortic valve calcium score (AVCS) and PVL [odds ratio (OR; per AVCS of 1000), 11.38; 95% confidence interval (CI) 2.33–55.53; $p = 0.001$)]. The mean AVCS in patients without PVL ($n = 66$) was 2704 ± 151, 3804 ± 2739 ($p = 0.05$) in mild PVL ($n = 31$), and 7387 ± 1044 ($p = 0.002$) with PVL ($n = 4$). An increase of the Agatston calcium score with 100 HU is associated with increased risk for PVL (odds ratio 1.09; 95% confidence interval 1.01–1.17; $p = 0.029$) [25].

– Bicuspid Aortic Valve
Bicuspid aortic valve (BAV) phenotype (Fig. 9.6) is the most common congenital valvular abnormality, occurring in 0.5–2% of the general population [28], and is associated with accelerated valve degeneration. BAV has so far been an exclusion criterion in randomized TAVI trials, so limited data about TAVI in BAV is available [1, 2]. TAVI in BAV may suffer from uneven frame expansion and subpar function, including PVL [29]. A systematic review on TAVI in BAV reported a 31% incidence of ≥ moderate PVL [30]. The rate of at least moderate PVL post TAVI seems consistently higher with BAV vs. tricuspid aortic stenosis (25% vs. 15%, $p = 0.05$) [31]. BAV tends to have a higher degree of root calcification (Agatston score 1262.7 ± 396.0 vs. 556.4 ± 461.9, $p < 0.01$) [32]. The self-expandable Medtronic CoreValve seems more underexpanded in BAV than

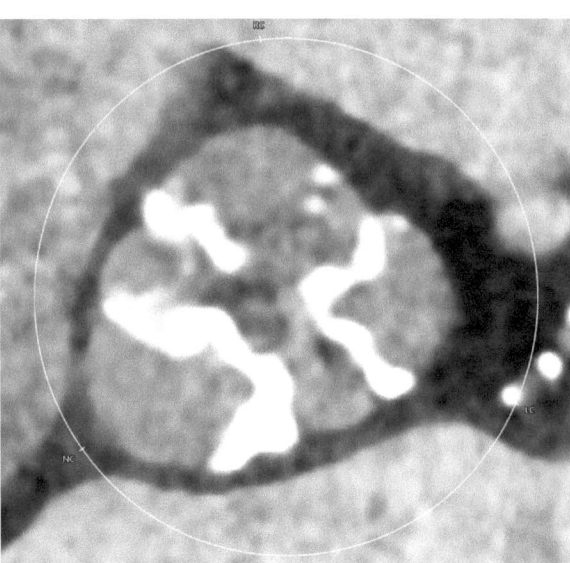

Fig. 9.5 MSCT image of a severely calcified tricuspid aortic valve. *NC* noncoronary cusp, *RC* right coronary cusp, *LC* left coronary cusp

Fig. 9.6 MSCT image of a
calcified bicuspid aortic
valve type I L-R, with
fusion of the left and
right coronary cusp.
NC noncoronary cusp,
RC right coronary cusp,
LC left coronary cusp

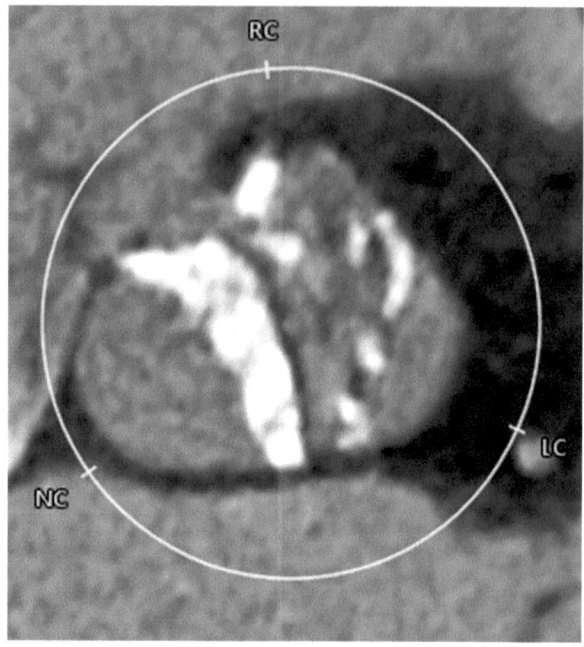

in degenerated tricuspid aortic valves (underexpansion at base of the stent frame
in $81.7\% \pm 14.9\%$ vs. $94.7\% \pm 15.0\%$, $p = 0.06$; at annulus level, $74.3\% \pm 16.7\%$
vs. $89.9\% \pm 10.5\%$, $p = 0.03$; at leaflet level, $64.6\% \pm 13.1\%$ vs. $81.2\% \pm 13.2\%$,
$p < 0.01$) [32].

9.3.2 Procedural Factors

– Valve Type
  Several meta-analyses suggest that the frequency of PVL is higher with self-
  expandable valves (SEV) than with the balloon-expandable valves (BEV) [7, 33].
  In the randomized Comparison of Transcatheter Heart Valves in High-Risk Patients
  With Severe Aortic Stenosis: Medtronic CoreValve Versus Edwards SAPIEN XT
  (CHOICE) trial, PVL assessed by contrast aortography and TTE was more fre-
  quent with Medtronic CoreValve SEV as compared to SAPIEN XT [34]. The niti-
  nol SEV frame has lower radial force than the stainless steel BAV frame [35]
  which may explain a more ellipsoid and underexpanded frame configuration with
  SEV by rotational angiography and a higher incidence of $\geq$ moderate PVL [36].

– Patient Prosthesis Mismatch
  Sizing for TAVI relies on a detailed aortic root assessment by noninvasive imaging techniques. Oversizing relative to the native annulus may provoke conduction abnormalities or more rarely annulus rupture and coronary obstruction,
  whereas undersizing may increase the risk for valve embolization and PVL.

Three-dimensional, volume-rendered multi-sliced computed tomography (MSCT) is currently "the gold standard" for aortic annulus measurement and device sizing. Echocardiography typically underestimates annular dimensions and may thus predispose to valve undersizing and PVL [37, 38]. Indeed MSCT-guided annular sizing reduced the incidence of >mild PVL when compared with two-dimensional TEE-guided annular sizing (7.5% vs. 21.9%; $p = 0.045$) [38].

– Prosthesis Malpositioning
  Appropriate positioning of THV is essential. Various THVs have a sealing mechanism (i.e., skirt) (Fig. 9.7), located at the lower part of the frame, to minimize retrograde blood flow into the LV. However, in too deep implantations (too ventricular) (Fig. 9.8a), the sealing fabric ends up below the native annulus. In case of a too high (aortic) implantation (Fig. 9.8b), the THV may not cover the native annulus.

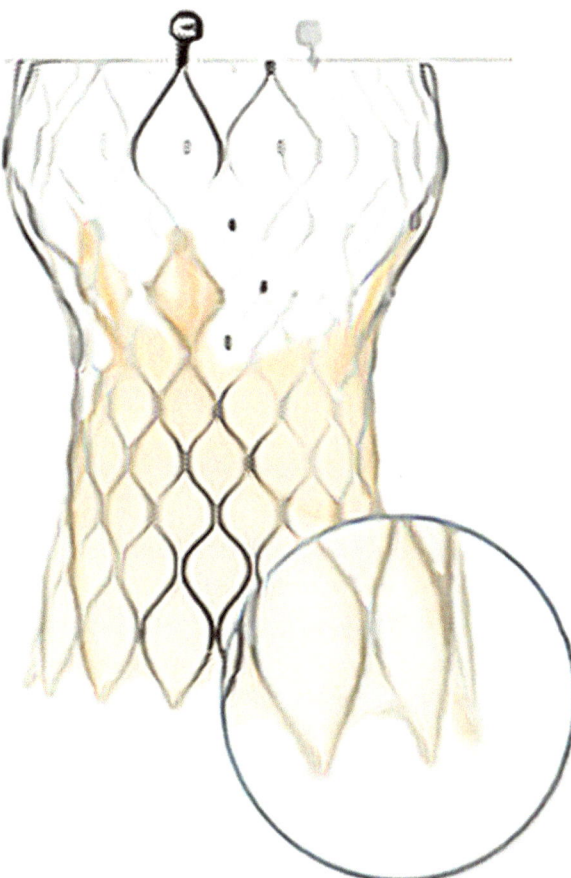

Fig. 9.7 Example of a sealing mechanism at the inflow portion of the frame of the transcatheter heart valve

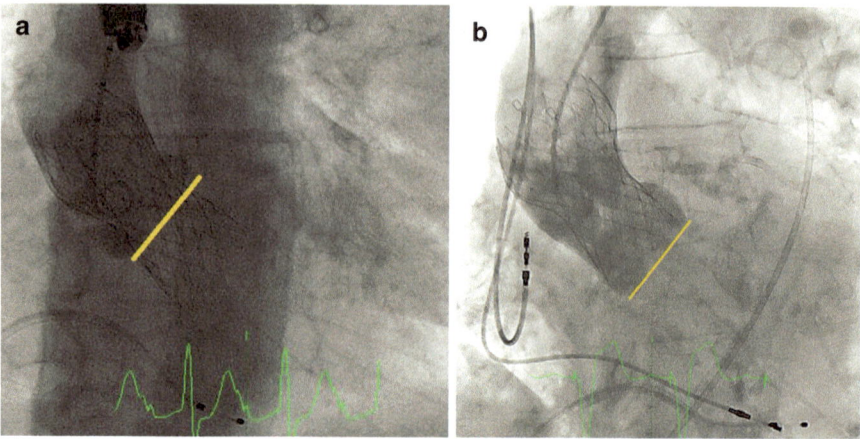

Fig. 9.8 Angiographic view of (**a**) a too deep (too ventricular) and (**b**) a too high (too aortic) implantation of a transcatheter aortic heart valve. *Yellow line*: native aortic annulus

9.3.3 Post-procedural Factor

9.3.3.1 Prosthetic Valve Endocarditis

Prosthetic valve endocarditis (PVE) is diagnosed according to the modified Duke criteria [39]. PVE is a rare but serious complication after TAVI, with an incidence varying in the literature from 0.6% to 3.4% [1, 40, 41]. A large multicenter registry reported a 1.13% PVE incidence [42]. PVE may damage the leaflets and/or framework and extend into paravalvular tissue causing AR (transvalvular and/or paravalvular). A multicenter study reported new or worsening AR in 15.1% of TAVI patients with PVE [43].

9.4 Treatment

9.4.1 Balloon Postdilatation

Balloon postdilatation may (partly) correct frame underexpansion (Fig. 9.9). Balloon postdilatation can improve frame expansion and reduce PVL in the majority of patients with ≥ moderate PVL [44].

However, balloon postdilatation may be associated with a higher risk for THV migration, trauma to the conduction system, rupture of the aortic annulus, and cerebrovascular embolism.

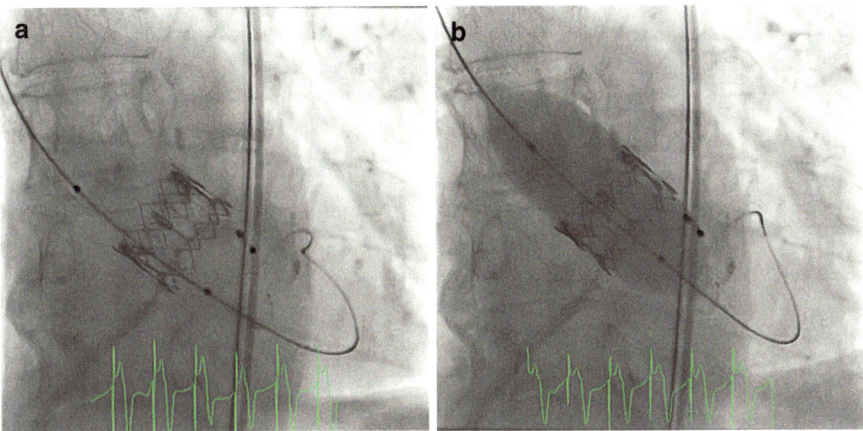

Fig. 9.9 Angiographic image of (**a** + **b**) post-balloon dilatation in a transcatheter heart valve

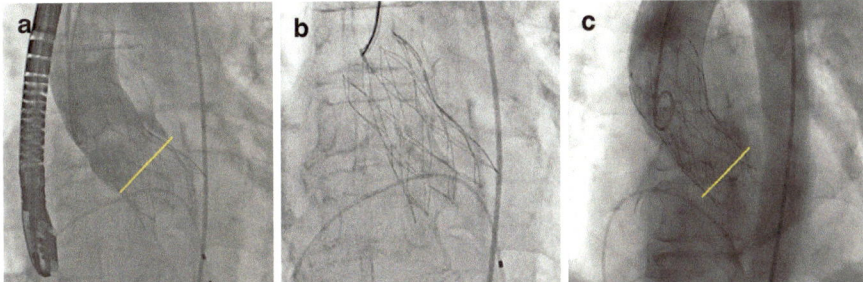

Fig. 9.10 Angiographic image of (**a**) a too deep implantation of transcatheter heart valve (**b**) snare catheter is engaged to the hook of the prosthesis (**c**) final corrected position of transcatheter heart valve. *Yellow line*: native aortic annulus.

9.4.2   Snaring

Snaring may correct valve malpositioning (Fig. 9.10). A snare catheter can be advanced through a femoral or radial/brachial approach. Potential risks of this maneuver are valve embolization, cerebral embolization, and aortic tear/dissection.

9.4.3   Valve in Valve

A viable treatment option for patients with a malpositioned valve (i.e., too deep or too high) is the valve-in-valve (VinV) technique. A second valve is then implanted several millimeters above or below the first malpositioned valve allowing the skirt of the stent frame to seal the native annulus (Fig. 9.11). In the Italian CoreValve registry, VinV technique was required in 24 of 663 patients (3.6%) [45]. The procedural 30-day and 12-month outcome of the VinV group was not different from the no-VinV group. VinV was safe with no impingement of the coronary ostia, embolic events, or excess intra-procedural or 30-day mortality. Importantly no significant increase in transvalvular gradient was observed. At 12 months, PVL grade ≥ 2 was seen in 1 of the 24 patients (4.2%) in the VinV group [45]. Patients with VinV had a higher need for permanent pacemaker implantation (33.3% vs. 14.5%, $p = 0.020$) because in the majority of cases, the first THV had been implanted too deep [45, 46].

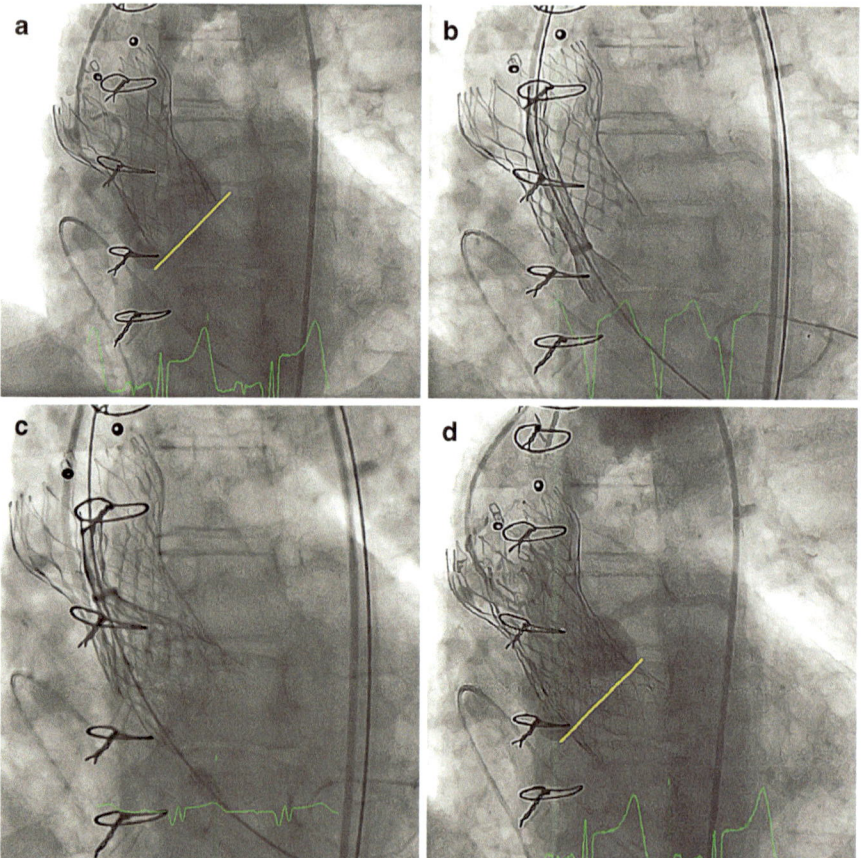

Fig. 9.11 Angiographic image of (**a**) a too high (too aortic) implantation of a transcatheter heart valve (THV), (**b** + **c**) implantation of a second valve several millimeters below the first THV. (**d**) Fully expanded second THV several millimeters below the native aortic annulus. *Yellow line*: native aortic annulus

9.4.4   Percutaneous Closure with a Plug

Vascular plugs can be used for percutaneous closure of PVL (off label). The implantation of the vascular plug is generally performed under fluoroscopy with or without TEE guidance. Briefly, the PVL is crossed with wire and catheter. The plug is then advanced to fill the periprosthetic space. A systematic review on this technique confirmed a relatively high success rates (86.9%) with both self-expandable and balloon-expandable THVs (100% vs. 77.8%, $p = 0.095$) [46]. Valve embolization occurred in one patient [47].

9.5   New Technologies

9.5.1   Second-Generation Valves

Second-generation valves (Fig. 9.12) introduce repositionability/retrievability, sealing fabric and/or frame adjustments to address the limitations of first generation valves (e.g., PVL). THV repositionability may improve overall THV positioning. So far repositioning with these next-generation THVs seems a safe concept. Notably, no excess in cerebrovascular events was reported [48]. In a propensity-matched analysis ≥ moderate, PVL was more frequent with first-generation THVs vs. second-generation THVs (17.5% vs. 5.8%; odds ratio, 0.30; 95% CI, 0.13–0.69; $p < 0.001$) with no difference in 30-day all-cause mortality (5.2% vs. 3.2%; odds ratio, 0.61; 95% CI, 0.20–1.92; $p = 0.40$) [49].

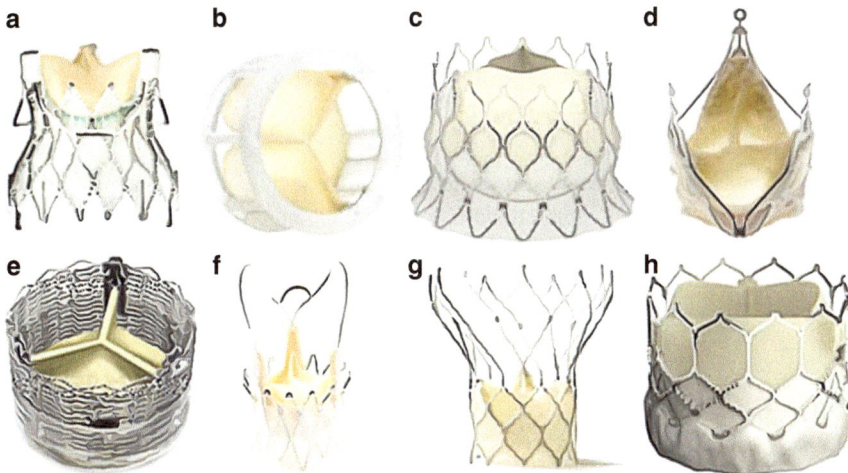

Fig. 9.12 Second-generation transcatheter aortic heart valves: (**a**) Engager valve, (**b**) Direct Flow, (**c**) Edwards Centera valve, (**d**) JenaValve, (**e**) Lotus Valve, (**f**) Symetis ACURATE, (**g**) Portico valve, (**h**) Edwards SAPIEN 3 valve

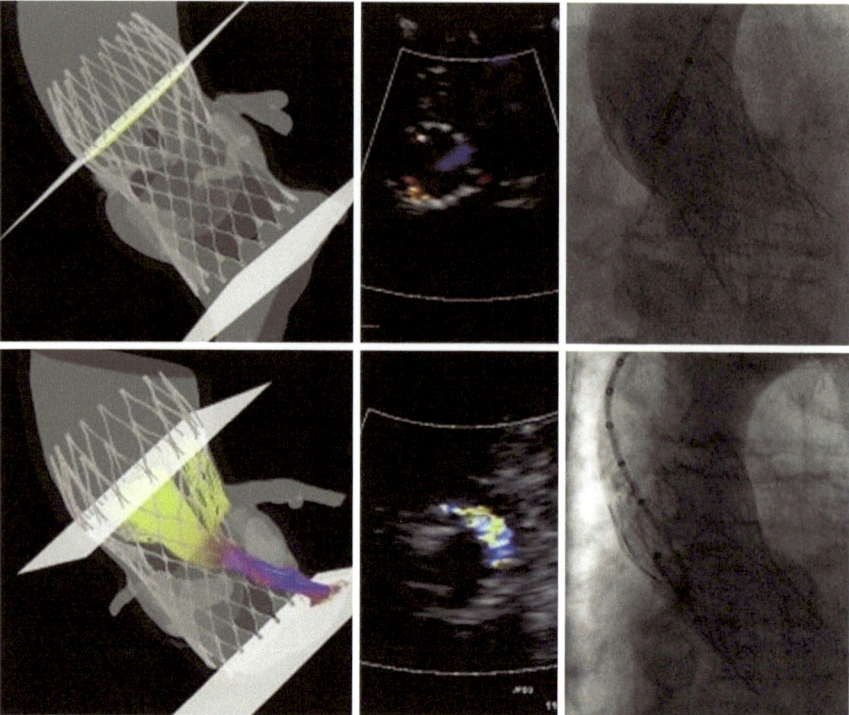

Fig. 9.13 *Top row*: example of a prediction model of a patient in which no PVL was predicted corresponding well with echocardiography and angiography (both grade 0). *Bottom row*: example of a prediction model of a patient in which PVL of 16 ml/s was predicted corresponding well with echocardiography (grade 2) and angiography (grade 3). Image courtesy of Prof. Dr. Peter de Jaegere, MD, PhD; Department of Cardiology, Erasmus Medical Center

9.5.2   THV Simulation

MSCT datasets can be used to simulate and predict device-host interactions by performing a virtual THV implantation in a 3D annular reconstruction. Simulation models accurately predicted calcium displacements and final PVL location and severity [50, 51] (Fig. 9.13). This concept can help determine the optimal valve size and implantation depth and support a true patient-tailored approach in the future.

9.6   Conclusion

The issue of paravalvular leakage with TAVI has multiple dimensions. Where challenges in accurate assessment and treatment remain, current-generation transcatheter heart valve technology experience and improved implantation techniques have dramatically reduced PVL frequency, making TAVI a valid treatment for a growing number of patients justifying extended adoption in clinical practice.

References

1. Smith CR, Leon MB, Mack MJ, Miller DC, Moses JW, Svensson LG, et al. Transcatheter versus surgical aortic-valve replacement in high-risk patients. N Engl J Med. 2011;364(23):2187–98. doi:10.1056/NEJMoa1103510. Epub 2011 Jun 5
2. Leon MB, Smith CR, Mack M, Miller DC, Moses JW, Svensson LG, et al., PARTNER Trial Investigators. Transcatheter aortic-valve implantation for aortic stenosis in patients who cannot undergo surgery. N Engl J Med. 2010;363(17):1597–607. doi:10.1056/NEJMoa1008232. Epub 2010 Sep 22
3. Leon MB, Smith CR, Mack MJ, Makkar RR, Svensson LG, Kodali SK, et al., PARTNER 2 Investigators. Transcatheter or surgical aortic-valve replacement in intermediate-risk patients. N Engl J Med . 2016;374(17):1609–20. doi:10.1056/NEJMoa1514616. Epub 2016 Apr 2
4. Kodali SK, Williams MR, Smith CR, Svensson LG, Webb JG, Makkar RR, et al., PARTNER Trial Investigators. Two-year outcomes after transcatheter or surgical aortic-valve replacement. N Engl J Med. 2012;366(18):1686–95. doi:10.1056/NEJMoa1200384. Epub 2012 Mar 26
5. Tamburino C, Capodanno D, Ramondo A, Petronio AS, Ettori F, Santoro G, et al. Incidence and predictors of early and late mortality after transcatheter aortic valve implantation in 663 patients with severe aortic stenosis. Circulation. 2011;123(3):299–308. doi:10.1161/CIRCULATIONAHA.110.946533. Epub 2011 Jan 10
6. Takagi H, Umemoto T, ALICE (All-Literature Investigation of Cardiovascular Evidence) Group. Impact of paravalvular aortic regurgitation after transcatheter aortic valve implantation on survival. Int J Cardiol. 2016;221:46–51. doi:10.1016/j.ijcard.2016.07.006. [Epub ahead of print]
7. Athappan G, Patvardhan E, Tuzcu EM, Svensson LG, Lemos PA, Fraccaro C, et al. Incidence, predictors, and outcomes of aortic regurgitation after transcatheter aortic valve replacement: meta-analysis and systematic review of literature. J Am Coll Cardiol. 2013;61:1585–95.
8. Sellers RD, Levy MJ, Amplatz K, Lillehey CW. Left retorgrade cardioangiography in acquired cardiac disease: technic, indications and interpretations in 700 cases. Am J Cardiol. 1964;14:437–47.
9. Schultz CJ, Slots TL, Yong G, Aben JP, Van Mieghem N, Swaans M, et al. An objective and reproducible method for quantification of aortic regurgitation after TAVI. EuroIntervention. 2014;10(3):355–63. doi:10.4244/EIJY14M05_06.
10. Tateishi H, Campos CM, Abdelghani M, Leite RS, Mangione JA, Bary L, et al. Video densitometric assessment of aortic regurgitation after transcatheter aortic valve implantation: results from the Brazilian TAVI registry. EuroIntervention. 2016;11(12):1409–18. doi:10.4244/EIJV11I12A271.
11. Sinning JM, Hammerstingl C, Vasa-Nicotera M, Adenauer V, Lema Cachiguango SJ, Scheer AC, et al. Aortic regurgitation index defines severity of peri-prosthetic regurgitation and predicts outcome in patients after transcatheter aortic valve implantation. J Am Coll Cardiol. 2012;59(13):1134–41. doi:10.1016/j.jacc.2011.11.048.
12. Jilaihawi H, Kar S, Doctor N, Fontana G, Makkar R. Contemporary application of cardiovascular hemodynamics: transcatheter aortic valve interventions. Cardiol Clin. 2011;29(2):211–22. doi:10.1016/j.ccl.2011.01.002.
13. Sinning JM, Stundl A, Pingel S, Weber M, Sedaghat A, Hammerstingl C, et al. Pre-procedural hemodynamic status improves the discriminatory value of the aortic regurgitation index in patients undergoing transcatheter aortic valve replacement. JACC Cardiovasc Interv. 2016;9(7):700–11. doi:10.1016/j.jcin.2015.12.271.
14. Höllriegel R, Woitek F, Stativa R, Mangner N, Haußig S, Fuernau G, et al. Hemodynamic assessment of aortic regurgitation after transcatheter aortic valve replacement: the diastolic pressure-time index. JACC Cardiovasc Interv. 2016;9(10):1061–8. doi:10.1016/j.jcin.2016.02.012. Epub 2016 Apr 27

15. Kappetein AP, Head SJ, Généreux P, Piazza N, van Mieghem NM, Blackstone EH, et al., Valve Academic Research Consortium-2. Updated standardized endpoint definitions for transcatheter aortic valve implantation: the Valve Academic Research Consortium-2 consensus document. J Thorac Cardiovasc Surg. 2013;145(1):6–23. doi:10.1016/j.jtcvs.2012.09.002. Epub 2012 Oct 16
16. Orwat S, Diller GP, Kaleschke G, Kerckhoff G, Kempny A, Radke RM, et al. Aortic regurgitation severity after transcatheter aortic valve implantation is underestimated by echocardiography compared with MRI. Heart. 2014;100(24):1933–8. doi:10.1136/heartjnl-2014-305665. Epub 2014 Jul 24
17. Crouch G, Tully PJ, Bennetts J, Sinhal A, Bradbrook C, Penhall AL, et al. Quantitative assessment of paravalvular regurgitation following transcatheter aotic valve. J Cardiovasc Magn Reson. 2015;17:32. doi:10.1186/s12968-015-0134-0.
18. Geleijnse ML, Di Martino LF, Vletter WB, Ren B, Galema TW, Van Mieghem NM, et al. Limitations and difficulties of echocardiographic short-axis assessment of paravalvular leakage after corevalve transcatheter aortic valve implantation. Cardiovasc Ultrasound. 2016;14(1):37. doi:10.1186/s12947-016-0080-5.
19. Van Belle E, Rauch A, Vincent F, Robin E, Kibler M, Labreuche J, et al. Von Willebrand factor multimers during transcatheter aortic-valve replacement. N Engl J Med. 2016;375(4):335–44. doi:10.1056/NEJMoa1505643.
20. Van Mieghem NM, Schultz CJ, van der Boon RM, Nuis RJ, Tzikas A, Geleijnse ML, et al. Incidence, timing, and predictors of valve dislodgment during TAVI with the Medtronic Corevalve System. Catheter Cardiovasc Interv. 2012;79(5):726–32. doi:10.1002/ccd.23275. Epub 2011 Dec 12
21. Ewe SH, Ng AC, Schuijf JD, van der Kley F, Colli A, Palmen M, et al. Location and severity of aortic valve calcium and implications for aortic regurgitation after transcatheter aortic valve implantation. Am J Cardiol. 2011;108(10):1470–7. doi:10.1016/j.amjcard. 2011.07.007. Epub 2011 Aug 17
22. Colli A, D'Amico R, Kempfert J, Borger MA, Mohr FW, Walther T. Transesophageal echocardiographic scoring for transcatheter aortic valve implantation: impact of aortic cusp calcification on postoperative aortic regurgitation. J Thorac Cardiovasc Surg. 2011;142(5):1229–35. doi:10.1016/j.jtcvs.2011.04.026.
23. Koos R, Mahnken AH, Dohmen G, Brehmer K, Günther RW, Autschbach R, et al. Association of aortic valve calcification severity with the degree of aortic regurgitation after transcatheter aortic valve implantation. Int J Cardiol. 2011;150(2):142–5. doi:10.1016/j.ijcard.2010.03.004. Epub 2010 Mar 28
24. Di Martino LFM, Vletter WB, Ren B, Schultz C, Van Mieghem NM, Soliman OII, et al. Prediction of paravalvular leakage after transcatheter aortic valve implantation. Int J Cardiovasc Imaging. 2015;31(7):1461–8.
25. Unbehaun A, Pasic M, Dreysse S, Drews T, Kukucka M, Mladenow A, et al. Transapical aortic valve implantation: incidence and predictors of paravalvular leakage and transvalvular regurgitation in a series of 358 patients. J Am Coll Cardiol. 2012;59(3):211–21. doi:10.1016/j. jacc.2011.10.857.
26. Pavicevic J, Nguyen TD, Caliskan E, Reser D, Frauenfelder T, Plass A, et al. Aortic valve calcium score is a significant predictor for the occurrence of post interventional paravalvular leakage after transcatheter aortic valve implantation. Results from a single center analysis of 260 consecutive patients. Int J Cardiol. 2015;181:185–7. doi:10.1016/j.ijcard.2014.12.032. Epub 2014 Dec 3
27. Haensig M, Lehmkuhl L, Rastan AJ, Kempfert J, Mukherjee C, Gutberlet M, et al. Aortic valve calcium scoring is a predictor of significant paravalvular aortic insufficiency in transapical-aortic valve implantation. Eur J Cardiothorac Surg. 2012;41(6):1234–1240.; discussion 1240–1. doi:10.1093/ejcts/ezr244. Epub 2012 Jan 12
28. Siu SC, Silversides CK. Bicuspid aortic valve disease. J Am Coll Cardiol. 2010;55:2789–800.

29. Zegdi R, Ciobotaru V, Noghin M, Sleilaty G, Lafont A, Latrémouille C, et al. Is it reasonable to treat all calcified stenotic aortic valves with a valved stent? Results from a human anatomic-study in adults. J Am Coll Cardiol. 2008;51(5):579–84. doi:10.1016/j.jacc.2007.10.023.
30. Yousef A, Simard T, Pourdjabbar A, Webb J, So D, Chong AY, et al. Performance of trans-catheter aortic valve implantation in patients with bicuspid aortic valve: systematic review. Int J Cardiol. 2014;176(2):562–4. doi:10.1016/j.ijcard.2014.07.013. Epub 2014 Jul 11
31. Bauer T, Linke A, Sievert H, Kahlert P, Hambrecht R, Nickenig G, et al. Comparison of the effectiveness of transcatheter aortic valve implantation in patients with stenotic bicuspid ver-sus tricuspid aortic valves (from the German TAVI Registry). Am J Cardiol. 2014;113(3):518–21. doi:10.1016/j.amjcard.2013.10.023. Epub 2013 Nov 9
32. Watanabe Y, Chevalier B, Hayashida K, Leong T, Bouvier E, Arai T, et al. Comparison of mul-tislice computed tomography findings between bicuspid and tricuspid aortic valves before and after transcatheter aortic valve implantation. Catheter Cardiovasc Interv. 2015;86(2):323–30. doi:10.1002/ccd.25830. Epub 2015 Feb 17
33. O'Sullivan KE, Gough A, Segurado R, Barry M, Sugrue D, Hurley JI. valve choice a sig-nificant determinant of paravalvular leak post-transcatheter aortic valve implantation? A sys-tematic review and meta-analysis. Eur J Cardiothorac Surg. 2014;45(5):826–33. doi:10.1093/ejcts/ezt515. Epub 2013 Nov 1
34. Abdel-Wahab M, Mehilli J, Frerker C, Neumann FJ, Kurz T, Tölg R, et al., CHOICE Investigators. Comparison of balloon-expandable vs self-expandable valves in patients undergoing transcatheter aortic valve replacement: the CHOICE randomized clinical trial. JAMA. 2014;311(15):1503–14. doi:10.1001/jama.2014.3316.
35. Tzamtzis S, Viquerat J, Yap J, Mullen MJ, Burriesci G. Numerical analysis of the radial force produced by the Medtronic-CoreValve and Edwards-SAPIEN after transcatheter aortic valve implantation (TAVI). Med Eng Phys. 2013;35(1):125–30.
36. Rodríguez-Olivares R, Rahhab Z, Faquir NE, Ren B, Geleijnse M, Bruining N, et al. Differences in frame geometry between balloon-expandable and self-expanding transcatheter heart valves and association with aortic regurgitation. Rev Esp Cardiol (Engl Ed). 2016;69(4):392–400. doi:10.1016/j.rec.2015.08.010. Epub 2015 Nov 28
37. Ng AC, Delgado V, van der Kley F, Shanks M, van de Veire NR, Bertini M, et al. Comparison of aortic root dimensions and geometries before and after transcatheter aortic valve implantation by 2- and 3-dimensional transesophageal echocardiography and multislice computed tomogra-phy. Circ Cardiovasc Imaging. 2010;3(1):94–102. doi:10.1161/CIRCIMAGING.109.885152. Epub 2009 Nov 17
38. Jilaihawi H, Kashif M, Fontana G, Furugen A, Shiota T, Friede G, et al. Cross-sectional com-puted tomographic assessment improves accuracy of aortic annular sizing for transcatheter aortic valve replacement and reduces the incidence of paravalvular aortic regurgitation. J Am Coll Cardiol. 2012;59(14):1275–86. doi:10.1016/j.jacc.2011.11.045. Epub 2012 Feb 22
39. Li JS, Sexton DJ, Mick N, Nettles R, Fowler VG Jr, Ryan T, et al. Proposed modifications to the duke criteria for the diagnosis of infective endocarditis. Clin Infect Dis. 2000;30(4):633–8. Epub 2000 Apr 3
40. Généreux P, Head SJ, Van Mieghem NM, Kodali S, Kirtane AJ, Xu K, et al. Clinical out-comes after transcatheter aortic valve replacement using valve academic research consortium definitions: a weighted meta-analysis of 3,519 patients from 16 studies. J Am Coll Cardiol. 2012;59:2317–26. doi:10.1016/j.jacc.2012.02.022.
41. Puls M, Eiffert H, Hünlich M, Schöndube F, Hasenfuß G, Seipelt R, et al. Prosthetic valve endo-carditis after transcatheter aortic valve implantation: the incidence in a single-centre cohort and reflections on clinical, echocardiographic and prognostic features. EuroIntervention. 2013;8:1407–18. doi:10.4244/EIJV8I12A214.
42. Latib A, Naim C, De Bonis M, Sinning JM, Maisano F, Barbanti M, et al. TAVR-associated prosthetic valve infective endocarditis: results of a large, multicenter registry. J Am Coll Cardiol. 2014;64(20):2176–8. doi:10.1016/j.jacc.2014.09.021. Epub 2014 Nov 10

43. Amat-Santos IJ, Messika-Zeitoun D, Eltchaninoff H, Kapadia S, Lerakis S, Cheema AN, et al. Infective endocarditis after transcatheter aortic valve implantation: results from a large multicenter registry. Circulation. 2015;131(18):1566–74. doi:10.1161/ CIRCULATIONAHA.114.014089. Epub 2015 Mar 9
44. Watanabe Y, Hayashida K, Lefèvre T, Romano M, Hovasse T, Chevalier B, et al. Is post-dilatation useful after implantation of the Edwards valve? Catheter Cardiovasc Interv. 2015;85(4):667–76. doi:10.1002/ccd.25486. Epub 2014 Apr 4
45. Ussia GP, Barbanti M, Ramondo A, Petronio AS, Ettori F, Santoro G, et al. The valve-in-valve technique for treatment of aortic bioprosthesis malposition an analysis of incidence and 1-year clinical outcomes from the italian CoreValve registry. J Am Coll Cardiol. 2011;57(9):1062–8. doi:10.1016/j.jacc.2010.11.019.
46. Piazza N, Onuma Y, Jesserun E, Kint PP, Maugenest AM, Anderson RH, et al. Early and persistent intraventricular conduction abnormalities and requirements for pacemaking after percutaneous replacement of the aortic valve. JACC Cardiovasc Interv. 2008;1(3):310–6. doi:10.1016/j.jcin.2008.04.007.
47. Ando T, Takagi H, ALICE (All-Literature Investigation of Cardiovascular Evidence) Group. Percutaneous closure of paravalvular regurgitation after transcatheter aortic valve implantation: a systematic review. Clin Cardiol. 2016;39(10):608–14. doi:10.1002/clc.22569. [Epub ahead of print]
48. Athappan G, Gajulapalli RD, Tuzcu ME, Svensson LG, Kapadia SR. A systematic review on the safety of second-generation transcatheter aortic valves. A systematic review on the safety of second-generation transcatheter aortic valves. EuroIntervention. 2016;11(9):1034–43. doi:10.4244/EIJV11I9A211.
49. Ruparelia N, Latib A, Kawamoto H, Buzzatti N, Giannini F, Figini F, et al. A Comparison between first-generation and second-generation Transcatheter Aortic Valve Implantation (TAVI) devices: a propensity-matched single-center experience. J Invasive Cardiol. 2016;28(5):210–6.
50. Schultz C, Rodriguez-Olivares R, Bosmans J, Lefèvre T, De Santis G, Bruining N, et al. Patient-specific image-based computer simulation for the prediction of valve morphology and calcium displacement after TAVI with the Medtronic CoreValve and the Edwards SAPIEN valve. EuroIntervention. 2016;11(9):1044–52. doi:10.4244/EIJV11I9A212.
51. de Jaegere P, De Santis G, Rodriguez-Olivares R, Bosmans J, Bruining N, Dezutter T, et al. Patient-specific computer modeling to predict aortic regurgitation after transcatheter aortic valve replacement. JACC Cardiovasc Interv. 2016;9(5):508–12.

Chapter 10
Transcatheter Management of TAVI-Associated Paravalvular Leak

Sahil Khera, Hasan Ahmad, Gilbert Tang, and Vinayak Bapat

Transcatheter aortic valve implantation (TAVI) has become a widely accepted treatment for the management of patients with severe aortic stenosis who are deemed prohibitive or high risk for conventional surgical replacement [1]. As data continue to emerge on the safety and efficacy of TAVI in patients who are at intermediate or low surgical risk, the utilization of TAVI for symptomatic severe aortic stenosis patients will increase in the near future [2–6]. Over eight TAVI devices are available in Europe, but the only valves approved for use in the USA are the Edwards SAPIEN balloon-expandable valve (Edwards Lifesciences, Irvine, CA) and the Medtronic self-expanding Evolut R and classic CoreValve (Medtronic, Minneapolis, MN) [7]. The SAPIEN XT and the SAPIEN 3 valves are now approved for intermediate-surgical-risk patients.

In the next few years, TAVI will likely become the treatment of choice for calcific degenerative aortic stenosis in all but the lowest-risk patients. Management and prevention of TAVI-related complications will therefore be extremely important. One important complication associated with TAVI is paravalvular leak (PVL) post-implantation which is uncommon in surgical valve replacement [8]. PVL will be a major limiting factor for ensuring optimal outcomes as lower-risk patients undergo TAVI. Lesser calcified valves, bicuspid valves, and TAVI for primary aortic regurgi-

S. Khera, M.D. • H. Ahmad, M.D.
Division of Cardiology, Westchester Medical Center/New York Medical College, Valhalla, New York, USA

G. Tang, M.D., M.Sc., M.B.A., F.R.C.S.C.
Department of Cardiovascular Surgery, Icahn School of Medicine at Mount Sinai, New York, NY, USA

V. Bapat, M.S., F.R.C.S., C.Th. (✉)
Assistant Professor Cardiothroacic Surgery, New York Presbyterian Hospital, Columbia University Medical Centre, 177 Fort Washington Avenue, MHB 7GN-435, New York 10032, USA
e-mail: vnbapat@yahoo.com

© Springer Nature Singapore Pte Ltd. 2017
G. Smolka et al. (eds.), *Transcatheter Paravalvular Leak Closure*,
DOI 10.1007/978-981-10-5400-6_10

153

tation will pose additional challenges to reduce PVL. Older data have reported that up to 67% of patients developed trivial/mild and up to 20% developed moderate to severe aortic regurgitation post-TAVI [9]. However, data from the PARTNER (Placement of Aortic Transcatheter Valves) 2A trial show a ≥ moderate PVL rate of 8.0%, data from the PARTNER 2-S3 show a ≥ moderate PVL rate of 3.8%, and data from the CoreValve Evolut R trial show a ≥ moderate PVL rate of 3.4% at 30 days [2, 10, 11]. Similarly, the Lotus and Direct Flow valves show a <2% rate of moderate or greater PVL. Moderate or greater PVL has been consistently associated with poorer outcomes in the short, mid-, and long term [12–14]. A recent meta-analysis and data from the PARTNER trial suggest that even mild PVL may be associated with higher mortality [15].

Accurate assessment of PVL postimplantation provides long-term prognostic data and guides therapy. Standardized grading of PVL still needs to be addressed, and a recent analysis showed 15.9% of patients graded as moderate by one corelab would be graded as mild by another corelab consortium [16]. All imaging modalities (echocardiography, aortography, computerized tomography (CT), cardiac magnetic resonance imaging (MRI), and hemodynamic assessment) have been utilized for the diagnosis of PVL post-TAVI but suffer from lack of standardization and validity [9]. Echocardiography (TEE) and hemodynamic assessment (using the aortic regurgitation index or AR index) in combination may offer the best immediate assessment of PVL [17, 18]. In our center we perform multimodality imaging immediately post-TAVI using transthoracic or transesophageal echocardiography, aortography, and hemodynamic assessment. In equivocal cases further imaging studies are undertaken using transesophageal echocardiography, CT, or cardiac MRI. Patients are also followed with echocardiographic assessment at intervals guided by initial severity and symptoms.

Several factors contribute to post-TAVI PVL. These include anatomic features of the native aortic valve, the specific type of valve used, improper valve implantation, and improper preprocedural aortic annulus sizing.

Native aortic valve anatomic features primarily relate to the aortic annulus which is a virtual ring formed at the hinge points of the aortic leaflets. Excessive aortic annular calcification and eccentricity may predispose to higher PVL rates due to frame under-expansion or incomplete apposition [19]. Improper aortic valve implantation techniques that predispose to PVL are usually due to infra-skirt PVL from high positioning or supra-skirt PVL due to low positioning (in the SAPIEN 3 and Evolut R valves) (relative to the aortic annulus) . The type of device used may affect PVL rates. The latest-generation balloon-expandable Edwards SAPIEN 3 has an external polyethylene terephthalate (PET) outer skirt which is designed to minimize paravalvular leak. The latest-generation Medtronic self-expanding Evolut R valve has an extended sealing skirt and more conformable inflow to minimize PVL. However, the Medtronic self-expanding valves are associated with modestly higher rates of PVL compared to Edwards SAPIEN valves or the Lotus or True Flow Valves [17, 20–22]. Lastly, prevention of PVL may be easier than post-TAVI treatment of PVL. This is most easily achieved with accurate 3D CT or TEE-guided sizing of the aortic annulus which avoids PVL related to annulus prosthesis mismatch. Accurate annulus sizing and interrogation of the aortic valvular complex ensures precise over- or undersizing of specific types of valves based on annular area, aortic valvular complex dimensions, and most importantly calcification. This chapter focuses on the transcatheter management of paravalvular leaks (PVL) associated with TAVI.

10.1 Transcatheter Approaches

Intraoperative assessment of PVL post-valve implantation should provide information on the severity of aortic regurgitation, hemodynamic status, and the need for immediate corrective measures. The therapeutic decisions are sometimes difficult to make based on non-standardized methods of quantification, acute hemodynamic changes due to alternative causes, and known improvement of aortic regurgitation in patients on follow-up. The CoreValve Extreme Risk Pivotal Trial reported improvement in 82.8% of moderate PVLs (at discharge) on 12-month follow-up [23]. Therefore depending on the severity of PVL management, it may include (1) a wait and reassess approach, (2) post-dilatation, (3) placement of a second valve, and (4) placement of a vascular plug.

10.1.1 Wait and Reassess

In both balloon and self-expanding valves, there is evidence that PVL can improve significantly over a period of as little as 15–20 min [17]. In cases where the PVL grade is mild or intermediate between mild and moderate or where the risk of annular injury from balloon post-dilatation is high, watchful waiting may result in significant improvement in the PVL grade. Before proceeding with more aggressive treatment (such as balloon post-dilatation), a risk/benefit decision should be made weighing the risk of aortic root injury or device embolization against the consequences of persistent PVL.

10.1.2 Balloon Post-Dilation

Balloon post-dilation treats PVL from frame under-expansion usually from a heavily calcified valve (Fig. 10.1). Provided a patient has no high-risk features of aortic root injury (female sex, excessive annular or LVOT calcium, narrow sinotubular junction) or high risk of device embolization (high implant above annulus, undersized valve which appears unstable), balloon post-dilation can be performed safely [24, 25]. The aggressiveness of balloon post-dilation is usually based on the degree of initial valve oversizing or undersizing and risk of aortic root injury. For Medtronic CoreValve classic and Evolut R self-expanding valves, a balloon size equal to the

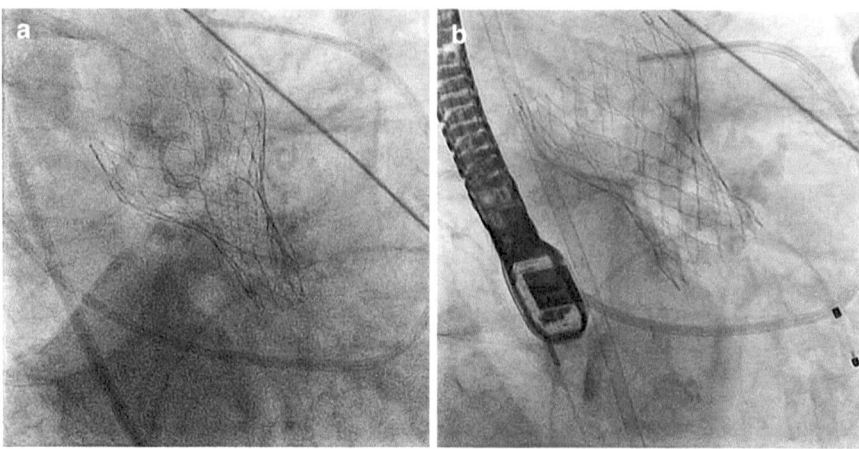

Fig. 10.1 Balloon post-dilation: under expanded Medtronic CoreValve after deployment with severe paravalvular leak (**a**), excellent results post-dilatation (**b**)

mean annular diameter is typically recommended (minus 1 mm if a less aggressive post-dilation is desired), and the balloon is positioned such that approximately 50% of the balloon length is above the valve inflow. A variety of balloon catheters in different sizes may be used. These included the semi-compliant Z-MED II™ Balloon Aortic Valvuloplasty catheters (B. Braun Interventional Systems, Bethlehem PA, USA), the non-compliant Bard True Balloon, or the newer Bard True Flow Balloon which allows continuous cardiac blood flow during balloon inflation via a central lumen. The InterValve V8 hourglass-shaped balloon has also been used to reduce PVL in self-expanding valves [26]. Post-dilation of the Edwards SAPIEN valve is usually performed using the initial valve deployment balloon by adding up to 2 cc extra volume in the inflation syringe and taking care to position the balloon slightly below the outflow to prevent flaring and overexpansion of the outflow [27].

Complications of balloon post-dilation include device migration/displacement, aortic wall injury/rupture, cerebrovascular events, and injury to the conduction system. Cerebrovascular events are an area of intense research as they can offset the hemodynamic benefits of post-dilation [28]. Initial reports by Nombela-Franco and coworkers reported post-dilation as a risk factor for acute (<24 h) cerebrovascular events (OR, 2.46; 95% CI, 1.07–5.67) [29]. Data from Italy on ~1300 balloon-expandable and self-expandable TAVIs reported balloon post-dilation in 19.8% (63% success rate) and no association with all-cause and cardiovascular mortality and cerebrovascular events at 1 year [30]. In a recent analysis of the PARTNER 1 trial with Edwards SAPIEN valve, post-dilation was associated with increased risk of early acute/subacute stroke (<7 days) (HR, 1.90 [95% CI, 1.03–3.50], $p = 0.041$), but not of late (>7 days) stroke [27]. The study also reported no excess 1 year mortality associated with post-dilation on multivariable risk adjustment. More recent data in self-expanding valves show significant improvement in moderate or greater PVL and excellent safety [31]. Balancing the risk of early stroke with appropriate patient selection should be considered before performing post-dilation.

10.1.3 Snare Maneuvers and Valve-in-Valve Implantation

In the SAPIEN 3 and Evolut R valves, valve malpositioning results in infra-skirt PVL from high positioning or supra-skirt PVL due to low positioning, and balloon post-dilation is typically not helpful in these cases. A valve-in-valve approach is the most common treatment. In rare instances, snaring and removing the self-expanding CoreValve system may be successful although fine repositioning is very difficult with the snare method [32–34]. Snares are either single (Amplatz GooseNeck™, Medtronic) or multiloop (EN Snare® Merit Medical Systems, Inc.) and come in different sizes. Improved traction has been reported with transbrachial approach and may be tried if transfemoral snare approach is unsuccessful [35]. If successfully snared the self-expanding CoreValve can usually be collapsed completely or partially into the delivery sheath but may need to be deployed in the ascending aorta. Caution should be exercised during snare as calcium debris may be dislodged into the arterial tree or aortic injury may inadvertently occur. A fully expanded but malpositioned SAPIEN valve is typically not easily snared, and this approach is not recommended. If snared, the SAPIEN valve is typically deployed in the aorta.

The goal of a valve-in-valve approach is to place the second valve incrementally higher or lower (depending on the original valve position) to provide the best sealing at the annulus and is the most common approach in cases of PVL due to malpositioning (Fig. 10.2).

Knowledge of the aortic complex dimensions is very important when attempting a valve-in-valve procedure. First an avoidable mechanism of malpositioning should be determined (septal bulge causing an upward displacement or VPC/suboptimal

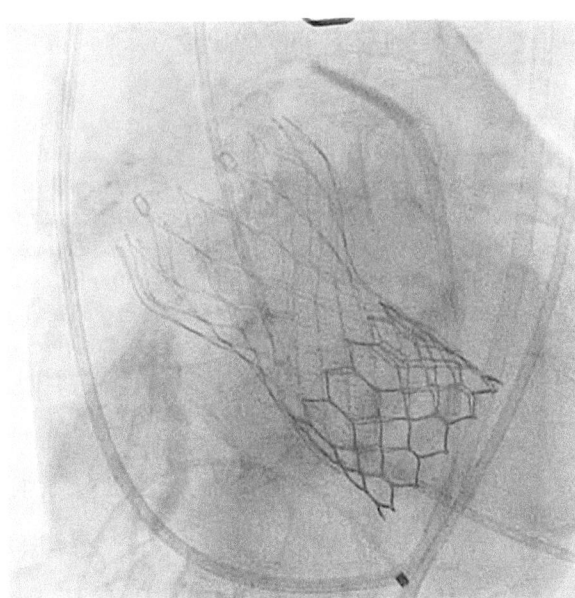

Fig. 10.2 Valve-in-valve: Worsening paravalvular leak 1 month post-Medtronic CoreValve implantation corrected with deployment of Edwards SAPIEN 3 valve-in-valve

rapid pacing causing valve displacement). Coronary occlusion is a potentially lethal complication of a valve-in-valve procedure and most likely to occur in a CoreValve that has been placed too low. When the second valve is placed higher inside the first valve, the leaflets of the original valve are displaced upward creating a "tube graft" and may cause coronary obstruction if the sinotubular junction is too narrow or the sinuses of Valsalva are small. Data from the Italian CoreValve Registry reported outcomes in 3.6% of patients undergoing valve-in-valve procedure for severe PVL pot conventional TAVI (75% with too low/ventricular placement and 25% with too high/supra-annular placement). They reported a procedural success in 98% of cases. At 1 year, the major adverse cardiac events were numerically higher but did not meet statistical significance (4.5% conventional TAVI versus 14.1% in valve-in-valve group, $p = 0.158$) [36]. In a series from Quebec Heart and Lung Institute, St. Paul's Hospital, and Cleveland Clinic, 90% success rate was reported for valve-in-valve TAVI for prosthesis malfunction/malposition [37]. At one-year follow-up, only one patient had residual moderate PVL with mild or none PVL in other cases. Mortality was higher at 30 days in the valve-in-valve group compared to TAVI group; however it did not meet statistical significance (14.3% versus 7.3%, $p = 0.23$). Survival at 1 year was comparable in both groups (76% in valve-in-valve group versus 78% in TAVI alone). This study included only the Edwards balloon-expandable systems. The authors described the approach of deploying the second valve 25–35% higher or lower relative to the stent frame height (depending on the initial malposition) using the similar valve size [37]. Data clearly underline the safety and feasibility of performing valve-in-valve procedures intraoperatively. It is also a viable therapeutic procedure for late onset valve degeneration or worsening PVL with time [38].

10.1.4   Transcatheter "Plugs"

Percutaneous vascular plugs can be implanted in scenarios where conventional techniques are not successful—for example, in patients with appropriate prosthesis implant height and incomplete apposition due to severe calcification with no improvement in PVL after post-dilation [39]. Transcatheter closures of paravalvular leaks were first reported in 1992 [40]. The first device used was the double-umbrella device by Rashkind and Cuaso [41]. Paravalvular leaks have complex anatomy with irregular serpiginous shape, and no dedicated plugs are available for this indication. Vascular plugs have been used to manage postsurgical valvular leaks. The issue with such complex anatomy is challenging wire manipulation and catheter crossing and inadequate sealing with self-expanding valves.

The most commonly employed transcatheter closure device for post-TAVI PVL has been Amplatzer Vascular Plugs (AVP, St. Jude Medical, St. Paul, MN, USA). AVP III is a self-expanding nitinol meshwork with oblong cross-sectional-shaped oval discs with enhanced stability and ability to recapture and reposition [42]. AVP IV has gained popularity recently due to lower crossing profile (4F catheters compared to minimum 6F for AVP III), narrow tapering ends that cause less damage to left ventricular outflow, and wide midbody that prevents device embolization. The limitation of lower-profile catheters is that large leaks cannot be sealed with single AVP IV as the maximum available device diameter is 8 mm (compared to 14 mm for AVP III) [43–46]. Device selection is based on adequate sizing, location, and characteristics (calcification, anatomic landmarks in proximity) of PVL. Multimodality imaging is sometimes needed for challenging PVL anatomy.

Complications of vascular plugs are device embolization, obstruction to coronary blood flow, prosthetic leaflet injury, and hemolysis. Vascular plugs have been safely and effectively used for balloon-expandable and self-expandable aortic valves [47–50].

10.2   Conclusions and Future Directions

PVL, post-TAVI, is a risk factor for poorer short-, medium-, and long-term outcomes. As indications expand for the utilization of TAVI, more emphasis needs to be placed on appropriate patient and device selection. Early recognition, hemodynamic consequences, and quantification of PVL are of paramount importance, especially in the immediate postimplantation period. Newer devices and novel imaging modalities will help decrease the incidence of PVL. In the interim, post-dilation, snare maneuvers, vascular plugs, and valve-in-valve are viable options in carefully selected patients with hemodynamically significant PVL post-procedure.

References

1. Nishimura RA, Otto CM, Bonow RO, et al. 2014 AHA/ACC guideline for the management of patients with valvular heart disease: executive summary: a report of the American College of Cardiology/American Heart Association Task Force on Practice Guidelines. J Am Coll Cardiol. 2014;63:2438–88.
2. Leon MB, Smith CR, Mack MJ, et al. Transcatheter or surgical aortic-valve replacement in intermediate-risk patients. N Engl J Med. 2016;374:1609–20.
3. Vahl TP, Kodali SK, Leon MB. Transcatheter aortic valve replacement 2016: a modern-day "through the looking-glass" adventure. J Am Coll Cardiol. 2016;67:1472–87.
4. Siontis GC, Praz F, Pilgrim T, et al. Transcatheter aortic valve implantation vs. surgical aortic valve replacement for treatment of severe aortic stenosis: a meta-analysis of randomized trials. Eur Heart J. 2016;37(47):3503–12.
5. Piazza N, Kalesan B, van Mieghem N, et al. A 3-center comparison of 1-year mortality outcomes between transcatheter aortic valve implantation and surgical aortic valve replacement on the basis of propensity score matching among intermediate-risk surgical patients. JACC Cardiovasc Interv. 2013;6:443–51.
6. Wenaweser P, Stortecky S, Schwander S, et al. Clinical outcomes of patients with estimated low or intermediate surgical risk undergoing transcatheter aortic valve implantation. Eur Heart J. 2013;34:1894–905.
7. Webb JG, Wood DA. Current status of transcatheter aortic valve replacement. J Am Coll Cardiol. 2012;60:483–92.

8. Lerakis S, Hayek SS, Douglas PS. Paravalvular aortic leak after transcatheter aortic valve replacement: current knowledge. Circulation. 2013;127:397–407.
9. Abdelghani M, Soliman OI, Schultz C, Vahanian A, Serruys PW. Adjudicating paravalvular leaks of transcatheter aortic valves: a critical appraisal. Eur Heart J. 2016;37(34):2627–44.
10. Kodali S, Thourani VH, White J, et al. Early clinical and echocardiographic outcomes after SAPIEN 3 transcatheter aortic valve replacement in inoperable, high-risk and intermediate-risk patients with aortic stenosis. Eur Heart J. 2016;37(28):2252–62.
11. Manoharan G, Walton AS, Brecker SJ, et al. Treatment of symptomatic severe aortic stenosis with a novel resheathable supra-annular self-expanding transcatheter aortic valve system. JACC Cardiovasc Interv. 2015;8(10):1359–67.
12. Kodali SK, Williams MR, Smith CR, et al. Two-year outcomes after transcatheter or surgical aortic-valve replacement. N Engl J Med. 2012;366:1686–95.
13. Gotzmann M, Korten M, Bojara W, et al. Long-term outcome of patients with moderate and severe prosthetic aortic valve regurgitation after transcatheter aortic valve implantation. Am J Cardiol. 2012;110:1500–6.
14. Tamburino C, Capodanno D, Ramondo A, et al. Incidence and predictors of early and late mortality after transcatheter aortic valve implantation in 663 patients with severe aortic stenosis. Circulation. 2011;123:299–308.
15. Kodali S, Pibarot P, Douglas PS, et al. Paravalvular regurgitation after transcatheter aortic valve replacement with the Edwards sapien valve in the PARTNER trial: characterizing patients and impact on outcomes. Eur Heart J. 2015;36:449–56.
16. Hahn RT, Pibarot P, Weissman NJ, Rodriguez L, Jaber WA. Assessment of paravalvular aortic regurgitation after transcatheter aortic valve replacement: intra-core laboratory variability. J Am Soc Echocardiogr. 2015;28(4):415–22.
17. Genereux P, Head SJ, Hahn R, et al. Paravalvular leak after transcatheter aortic valve replacement: the new Achilles' heel? A comprehensive review of the literature. J Am Coll Cardiol. 2013;61:1125–36.
18. Jilaihawi H, Chakravarty T, Shiota T, et al. Heart-rate adjustment of transcatheter haemodynamics improves the prognostic evaluation of paravalvular regurgitation after transcatheter aortic valve implantation. Euro Intervention. 2015;11(4):456–64.
19. Tang GH, Lansman SL, Cohen M, Spielvogel D, Cuomo L, Ahmad H, Dutta T. Transcatheter aortic valve replacement: current developments, ongoing issues, future outlook. Cardiol Rev. 2013;21(2):55–76.
20. Athappan G, Patvardhan E, Tuzcu EM, et al. Incidence, predictors, and outcomes of aortic regurgitation after transcatheter aortic valve replacement: meta-analysis and systematic review of literature. J Am Coll Cardiol. 2013;61:1585–95.
21. Nombela-Franco L, Ruel M, Radhakrishnan S, et al. Comparison of hemodynamic performance of self-expandable CoreValve versus balloon-expandable Edwards SAPIEN aortic valves inserted by catheter for aortic stenosis. Am J Cardiol. 2013;111:1026–33.
22. Moat NE, Ludman P, de Belder MA, et al. Long-term outcomes after transcatheter aortic valve implantation in high-risk patients with severe aortic stenosis: the U.K. TAVI (United Kingdom Transcatheter Aortic Valve Implantation) Registry. J Am Coll Cardiol. 2011;58:2130–8.
23. Popma JJ, Adams DH, Reardon MJ, et al. Transcatheter aortic valve replacement using a self-expanding bioprosthesis in patients with severe aortic stenosis at extreme risk for surgery. J Am Coll Cardiol. 2014;63:1972–81.
24. Takagi K, Latib A, Al-Lamee R, et al. Predictors of moderate-to-severe paravalvular aortic regurgitation immediately after CoreValve implantation and the impact of postdilatation. Catheter Cardiovasc Interv. 2011;78:432–43.
25. Schultz C, Rossi A, van Mieghem N, et al. Aortic annulus dimensions and leaflet calcification from contrast MSCT predict the need for balloon post-dilatation after TAVI with the Medtronic CoreValve prosthesis. Euro Intervention. 2011;7:564–72.

26. Latib A, Pedersen W, Maisano F, et al. Initial findings using the V8 hourglass-shaped valvuloplasty balloon for postdilatation in treating paravalvular leaks associated with transcatheter self-expanding aortic valve prosthesis. Catheter Cardiovasc Interv. 2016;87(7):1306–13.

27. Hahn RT, Pibarot P, Webb J, et al. Outcomes with post-dilation following transcatheter aortic valve replacement: the PARTNER I trial (placement of aortic transcatheter valve). JACC Cardiovasc Interv. 2014;7:781–9.

28. Stortecky S, Windecker S. Stroke: an infrequent but devastating complication in cardiovascular interventions. Circulation. 2012;126:2921–4.

29. Nombela-Franco L, Webb JG, de Jaegere PP, et al. Timing, predictive factors, and prognostic value of cerebrovascular events in a large cohort of patients undergoing transcatheter aortic valve implantation. Circulation. 2012;126:3041–53.

30. Barbanti M, Petronio AS, Capodanno D, et al. Impact of balloon post-dilation on clinical outcomes after transcatheter aortic valve replacement with the self-expanding CoreValve prosthesis. JACC Cardiovasc Interv. 2014;7:1014–21.

31. Harrison J, Hughes GC, Reardon MJ, et al. TCT-94 balloon post-dilation of the self-expanding CoreValve transcatheter aortic valve bioprosthesis: procedural results and in hospital outcomes from 3532 patients in the CoreValve US Pivotal and Continued Access Trials. J Am Coll Cardiol. 2015;66(15_S). doi:10.1016/j.jacc.2015.08.139.

32. Vavouranakis M, Vrachatis DA, Toutouzas KP, Chrysohoou C, Stefanadis C. "Bail out" procedures for malpositioning of aortic valve prosthesis (CoreValve). Int J Cardiol. 2010;145:154–5.

33. Vavuranakis M, Vrachatis D, Stefanadis C. CoreValve aortic bioprosthesis: repositioning techniques. JACC Cardiovasc Interv. 2010;3:565. author reply 6

34. Majunke N, Doss M, Steinberg DH, et al. How should I treat a misplaced self-expanding aortic bioprosthetic valve? EuroIntervention. 2010;6:537–42.

35. Hoffmann R, Rieck B, Dohmen G. Correction of CoreValve position using snare traction from a right brachial artery access. J Invasive Cardiol. 2010;22:E59–60.

36. Ussia GP, Barbanti M, Ramondo A, et al. The valve-in-valve technique for treatment of aortic bioprosthesis malposition an analysis of incidence and 1-year clinical outcomes from the italian CoreValve registry. J Am Coll Cardiol. 2011;57:1062–8.

37. Toggweiler S, Wood DA, Rodes-Cabau J, et al. Transcatheter valve-in-valve implantation for failed balloon-expandable transcatheter aortic valves. JACC Cardiovasc Interv. 2012;5:571–7.

38. Hammerstingl C, Nickenig G, Grube E. Treatment of a degenerative stenosed CoreValve((R)) aortic bioprosthesis by transcatheter valve-in-valve insertion. Catheter Cardiovasc Interv. 2012;79:748–55.

39. Sinning JM, Vasa-Nicotera M, Werner N, Nickenig G, Hammerstingl C. Interventional closure of paravalvular leakage after transcatheter aortic valve implantation. Eur Heart J. 2012;33:2498.

40. Hourihan M, Perry SB, Mandell VS, Keane JF, Rome JJ, Bittl JA, Lock JE. Transcatheter umbrella closure of valvular and paravalvular leaks. J Am Coll Cardiol. 1992;20:1371–7.

41. Rashkind WJ, Cuaso CC. Transcatheter closure of a patent ductus arteriosus: successful use in a 3.5 kg infant. Pediatr Cardiol. 1979;1:3–7.

42. Buellesfeld L, Meier B. Treatment of paravalvular leaks through interventional techniques. Multimed Man Cardiothorac Surg. 2011;924

43. Feldman T, Salinger MH, Levisay JP, Smart S. Low profile vascular plugs for paravalvular leaks after TAVR. Catheter Cardiovasc Interv. 2014;83:280–8.

44. Luu J, Ali O, Feldman TE, Price MJ. Percutaneous closure of paravalvular leak after transcatheter aortic valve replacement. JACC Cardiovasc Interv. 2013;6:e6–8.

45. Whisenant B, Jones K, Horton KD, Horton S. Device closure of paravalvular defects following transcatheter aortic valve replacement with the Edwards Sapien valve. Catheter Cardiovasc Interv. 2013;81:901–5.

46. Don CW, Dean LS. Have we found the ideal plug for post-TAVR paravalvular leaks? Catheter Cardiovasc Interv. 2014;83:289–90.

47. Gafoor S, Franke J, Piayda K, Lam S, Bertog S, Vaskelyte L, Hofmann I, Sievert H. Paravalvular leak closure after transcatheter aortic valve replacement with a self-expanding prosthesis. Catheter Cardiovasc Interv. 2014;84:147–54.
48. Poliacikova P, Hildick-Smith D. Paravalvular leak closure for persisting aortic regurgitation after implantation of the CoreValve transcatheter valve. Catheter Cardiovasc Interv. 2014;84:155–9.
49. Arri SS, Poliacikova P, Hildick-Smith D. Percutaneous paravalvular leak closure for symptomatic aortic regurgitation after CoreValve transcatheter aortic valve implantation. Catheter Cardiovasc Interv. 2015;85:657–64.
50. Dhoble A, Chakravarty T, Nakamura M, Abramowitz Y, Tank R, Mihara H, Mangat G, Jilaihawi H, Shiota T, Makkar R. Outcome of paravalvular leak repair after transcatheter aortic valve replacement with a balloon-expandable prosthesis. Catheter Cardiovasc Interv. 2017;89(3):462–8. doi:10.1002/ccd.26570.

Chapter 11
Complications of Transcatheter Paravalvular Leak Closure

Rafael Hirsch

11.1 Introduction

Closure of paravalvular leak is one of the most complex and demanding catheter-based structural heart disease interventions.

The patient population treated for this disorder is often of advanced age and with multiple comorbidities. Many have had several heart operations and suffer from congestive heart failure, chronic anemia requiring in some cases repeated blood transfusions, renal failure, pulmonary hypertension, cardiac arrhythmia, and more.

Taking into consideration the complexity of the procedure and the degree of sickness of the patients, the rate of complications from paravalvular leak closure is relatively low and reassuring, especially when compared to the results of surgical intervention, which is the alternative solution [1, 2]. Also, it appears that recent publications report far better results than the initial reports, with a much lower complication rate and better success rate [3–7]. The number of cases reported to date from all publications combined is still relatively small, and the confounders are so varied and versatile that it is not possible to quote a true incidence of the complications, and therefore this chapter will focus on their description and the recommended approach for eliminating or reducing their incidence.

Transcatheter paravalvular leak closure is not a uniform procedure. The valves treated can be mitral or aortic, mechanical or biological, and surgical or catheter based. The approach can be transseptal, transaortic, or trans-apical (surgical or percutaneous), with or without general anesthesia, with or without use of contrast

R. Hirsch, M.D.
Department of Cardiology, Adult Congenital Heart Unit, Rabin Medical Center—Beilinson Campus, Petah Tikva and Sackler School of Medicine, Tel Aviv University, Tel Aviv, Israel
e-mail: rafaelh@clalit.org.il

© Springer Nature Singapore Pte Ltd. 2017
G. Smolka et al. (eds.), *Transcatheter Paravalvular Leak Closure*,
DOI 10.1007/978-981-10-5400-6_11

material, and so on. Diverse devices are being used for paravalvular leak closure. Complication rate and type vary according to each of the abovementioned parameters.

In this chapter, a structured approach to complications of paravalvular leak closure will be used, based on the available literature and personal experience of the author.

11.2 Transseptal Puncture

Complications of transseptal puncture are well known and not specific for closure of paravalvular leaks.

The two feared complications of transseptal puncture are free wall or organ perforation and systemic embolization of thrombus or air.

The two cardiac structures that lie adjacent to the atrial septum, the aorta anteriorly and the coronary sinus infero-posteriorly, particularly when enlarged, e.g., due to drainage of a left persistent caval vein, are prone to perforation during transseptal puncture [8]. The free wall of the atria may also be perforated under certain circumstances, though in patients with a paravalvular leak the left atrium is usually enlarged and less likely to perforate. As long as the perforation is recognized on time, with only the tip of the needle across the wall, withdrawal of the needle will usually suffice, and the risk of tamponade is small. However, if the entire transseptal system including an 8 or 9F sheath has entered the wrong space, this should bring the procedure to an immediate halt, and cardiac surgeons must be consulted. The system should not be instinctively withdrawn, as it might be stopping extravasation of blood, thus preventing cardiac tamponade or hemorrhagic shock. A case report describes an elegant way to solve the problem percutaneously [9].

When first introduced, transseptal puncture was performed with fluoroscopy only. Because of the inherent risk of perforation when puncturing the septum without imaging, it was customary to advise against anticoagulation until the septum has been safely crossed.

Nowadays imaging techniques are often accompanying transseptal puncture. This is certainly true for closure of paravalvular leaks which is always performed with imaging, mainly transesophageal echocardiography (TEE) but sometimes intracardiac echocardiography (ICE). Performing the puncture under "vision" reduces the likelihood of inadvertent perforation to almost zero. On the other hand, transseptal puncture in these patients may be prolonged because of very dilated atria, foreign material in the septum, and the need to puncture at a prespecified site to facilitate leak closure. Without anticoagulation there is a chance of thrombus formation on the transseptal system (Fig. 11.1), and if not recognized before crossing, the clot may be introduced by the advancing transseptal sheath into the left atrium and embolize systemically. Therefore, routine anticoagulation at half dose is given after introduction of the femoral sheaths and completion of the dose after successful transseptal puncture.

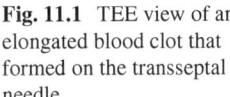

Fig. 11.1 TEE view of an elongated blood clot that formed on the transseptal needle

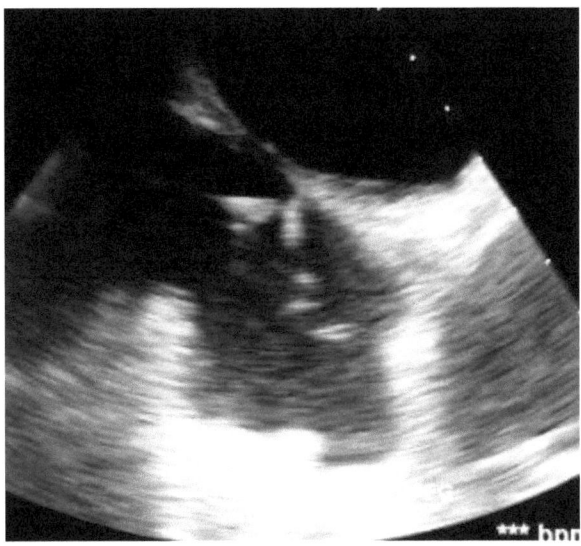

11.3   Complications of the Trans-apical Approach

The left ventricular apex can be used for PVL closure. It can be accessed through a surgical approach, performing a mini-thoracotomy in a hybrid catheterization laboratory, or percutaneously.

11.3.1   Surgical Trans-apical Approach

The majority of reports in the literature regarding a surgical transcatheter approach to structural interventions deal with valve implantations. These require very large sheaths and are not comparable in risk to PVL closure which requires much smaller sheaths and devices. In two series, 17 patients in one and seven in the other, the procedure was uneventful [2, 10], and in a third series, involving 37 patients, there were four cases of hemothorax requiring surgical re-thoracotomy. Procedure-related mortality occurred in one patient within 72 h and in two within 30 days [11].

At Rabin Medical Center, PVL closure through the apex is rarely performed and only through a surgical approach. There was one severe complication as follows:

Case No. 1

A 78-year-old gentleman presents with severe paravalvular mitral leak and advanced heart failure. The left ventricular apex was prepared with a purse-string suture very close to the ventricular septum, so that initial introduction of the sheath and wire

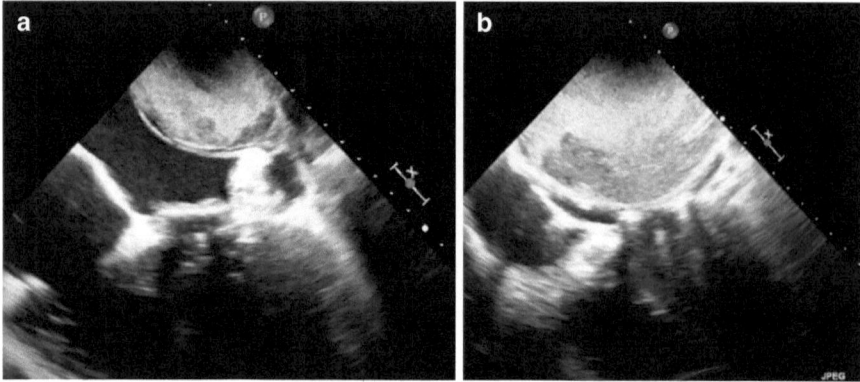

Fig. 11.2 Left atrial wall hematoma inside a dissection of the atrial wall caused by the wire while attempting to cross the leak. (**a**) Appearance at the cath. lab (**b**) Three days later, despite the appearance of the hematoma as if entirely obliterating the atrium and obstructing the valve, it had no clinical effect

was into the right ventricle. The sheath was pulled back and redirected toward the mitral valve ring, but most probably remained very close if not within the septum, so that when crossing the leak with a wire was attempted, a left atrial wall dissection occurred (Fig. 11.2). The procedure was abandoned, and the patient who was extremely sick prior to the procedure remained surprisingly stable for several days, despite the menacing appearance of the huge atrial wall hematoma that seemed to almost obliterate the left atrial chamber. However, he succumbed during a salvage operation.

11.3.2 Percutaneous Trans-apical Approach

The percutaneous approach has been used extensively by one group, led by Prof. Ruiz of New York. Complications include hemothorax, pericardial effusion and tamponade, coronary laceration, pneumothorax, cardiac arrhythmia, and death. There is potential for the development of left ventricular apical pseudoaneurysm.

Hemothorax is the most frequent complication. It can be related to coronary or intercostal vessel laceration or bleeding from the left ventricular puncture site. Coronary laceration can potentially be avoided with CT imaging guidance and coronary angiography when obtaining trans-apical access. A chest tube may be required for evacuation of the hematoma if the patient is symptomatic or difficult to ventilate. For cardiac tamponade, pericardial drainage is required with percutaneous drainage generally sufficient. However, emergent left lateral thoracotomy may be required to control access site bleeding, with intramyocardial placement of pledgeted sutures [12].

11.4 Access Site Complications

Access site complications are common to all percutaneous interventions, and the reporting of complications has become standardized by the VARC-2 definitions [13]. Access site complications of PVL closure are rare and usually mild, because most procedures are done transvenously, and arterial sheaths required rarely exceed 8F.

11.5 Wire Complications

11.5.1 Wire Perforation: Left Atrium

Having crossed the interatrial septum, efforts are directed toward crossing the leak. In leaks located directly at the orifice of the left atrial appendage, care should be taken not to introduce the catheter and wire inadvertently into the appendage, risking perforation of this relatively delicate organ. Focusing on the TEE image rather than fluoroscopy is key for preventing such complications.

Similarly, certain fluoroscopic angulations may superimpose structures, so that a wire that seems to cross a leak is actually in a completely different structure.

Case No. 2

An 82-year-old gentleman with severe paravalvular mitral leak had one device placed with what seemed as a significant residual leak. However, it was impossible to introduce a catheter over a second wire that was still across the leak, in order to implant a second device. The wire was removed in order to attempt recrossing the leak elsewhere. The wire could not be advanced properly into what was assumed to be the left ventricle. Also, it was not demonstrated on TEE and was therefore removed (Fig. 11.3a, b). It was decided to end the procedure with partial success.

However, when the patient was extubated, he had an immediate collapse, requiring resuscitation including cardiac massage. An urgent coronary arteriography demonstrated air bubbles in the coronary circulation and bypass grafts (Fig. 11.3c), and TEE showed air bubbles in the left atrium and accumulation of air at the LV apex (Fig. 11.3d). Within a few minutes, the patient's condition stabilized with recovery of blood pressure. A pigtail was introduced into the apex of the LV to evacuate as much of the accumulated air as possible. Recovery was uneventful. On the next day's echocardiogram, myocardial function was back to previous levels, and the residual leak was milder than expected (Fig. 11.3e).

It is assumed that on trying to recross the valve, the wire was inadvertently introduced into the left lower pulmonary vein and punctured it. Upon extubation and resumption of spontaneous breathing, air was sucked into the pulmonary vein causing this dramatic complication. Luckily, the puncture had sealed off within a few minutes, and normal circulation was restored.

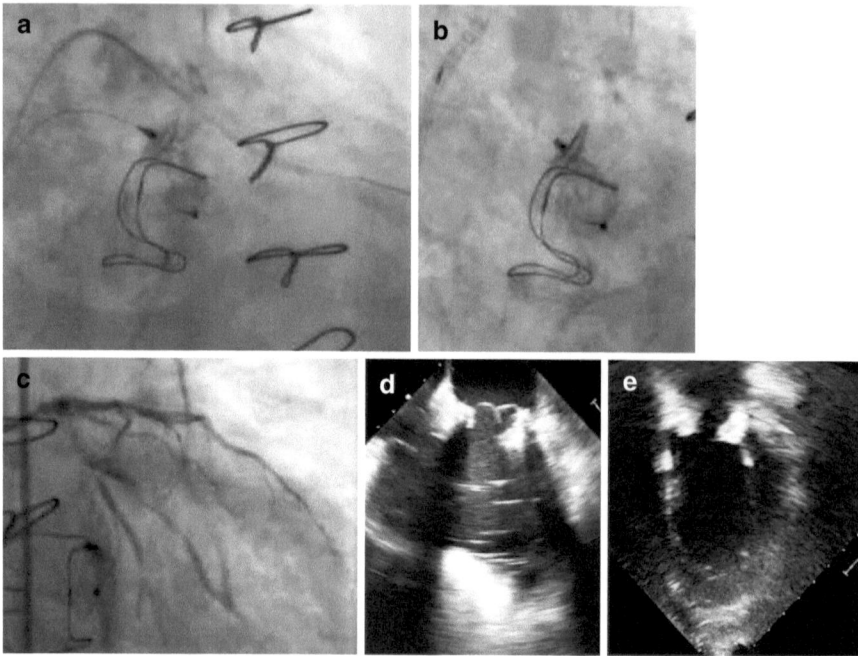

Fig. 11.3 (**a**) Fluoroscopy showing passage of catheter on wire parallel to the original device, assuming the leak was recrossed. (**b**) The catheter could not be seen on TEE and was withdrawn. The first device was released. (**c**) Collapse on extubation. Urgent coronary angiography shows air bubbles in coronary circulation. (**d**) TEE shows accumulation of air in the LV apex. (**e**) After a short resuscitation, the patient stabilized. On TEE the following day, no air remains, myocardial function restored to baseline, and the residual leak mild

Atrial wall wire perforation can occur when crossing the mitral valve leak retrogradely, entering the left ventricle from the aorta or through the apex. When it is chosen to "reverse sides" by creating a complete arterial venous wire loop, there will be a wire through the leak and a snare catheter through the transseptal puncture. The left atrium which is often dilated may make snaring challenging, and care should be taken when manipulating the wires to avoid perforation. When the retrograde approach for device placement is chosen, there is often a need to exchange for a stiffer wire, again with a risk of perforation of the atrial wall.

11.5.2 Wire Perforation: Left Ventricle

Crossing antegradely through a leak of the mitral valve or retrogradely through a leak of the aortic valve, there is potential for wire perforation of the left ventricular free wall. In order to reduce the risk of perforation, several precautions should be taken. Crossing the leak with a J-tipped hydrophyllic guidewire is preferable to a straight one. When the glidewire is replaced with a stiffer one to enable advancement of the sheath, wire position should be well secured while applying force against resistance of the often rough surface of the leak. Hydrophilic sheaths, e.g., Terumo Destination, enable smoother passage with less force applied on the system. Also, using several smaller devices enables the use of smaller sheaths with less resistance to crossing compared to a single large device. Finally, if the patient with para-mitral leak has a native aortic valve, performing a complete venous-arterial loop or even advancing the wire to the ascending aorta will reduce the risk of free wall myocardial perforation by the wire.

Case No. 3

A 65-year-old gentleman presents with para-aortic leak. The procedure was monitored with intracardiac echocardiography (ICE), and the patient was awake. At the time of advancing the sheath through the leak, over the extra-stiff wire, the patient complained of chest discomfort, and the whole system was immediately withdrawn. There were no ST changes on the monitor, and both on ICE and TTE, no pericardial effusion could be seen. As the symptoms subsided, the procedure was resumed, and a device was placed in the leak. Despite what was seemed a good seal of the leak, aortic regurgitation persisted, in a mechanism that was difficult to delineate. Therefore, several days later, the patient had a gated CT scan. On the CT scan, a wire perforation of the left ventricular apex was apparent, with accumulation of the blood only around the apex. This was treated conservatively and remained stable on a follow-up CT a week later. In patients who had several heart operations, there are multiple adhesions around the heart that may prevent cardiac tamponade from occurring after free wall puncture. It was the coincidence of an awake patient during the procedure, and a CT scan performed for another indication, that revealed this complication, which was initially suspected but then "ruled out" (Fig. 11.4).

11.5.3 Wire Entrapment

One case report describes entrapment of a wire introduced through a leak around an aortic valve bioprosthesis coming back through the valve to form an arterial-arterial wire loop. This required surgical removal [14].

11.6 Device-Related Complications

11.6.1 Leaflet Entrapment

An important factor in device-related complications is the type of valve. In mechanical valves, there is a risk of leaflet entrapment by the device [15, 16]. This is particularly true for the older single, tilting disk valves, e.g., the Bjork-Shiley.

Fig. 11.4 Wire perforation of the left ventricular apex during closure of aortic PVL, causing a very localized collection of blood, due to adhesions from repeated operations. The complication was suspected during the procedure when the patient complained of chest pain, but could not be confirmed. Only several days later, it was a coincidental finding of a CT scan ordered for evaluation of the residual leak

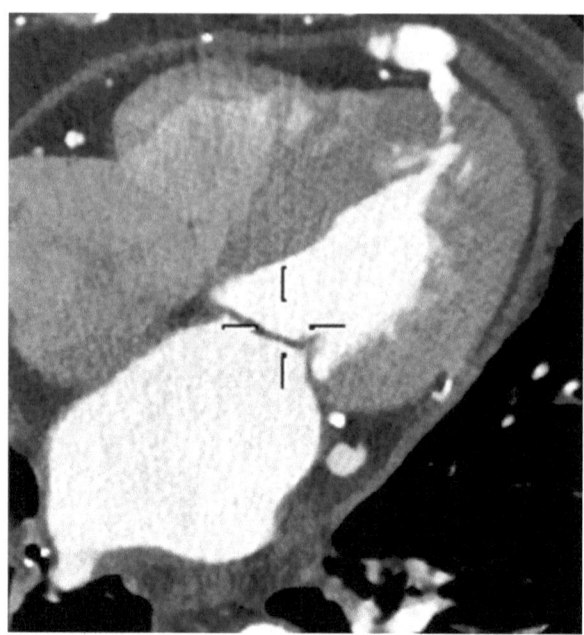

Much depends on the location of the leak in relation to the site of maximal protrusion of the disk from the valve ring. This of course cannot be changed, but prediction of a potential leaflet entrapment at the time of pre-procedure planning should be taken into account when choosing the type and size of device used and even the approach (antegrade vs. retrograde).

In general, smaller devices have less chance of catching valve leaflets. So moving from a single large device to multiple small devices may help prevent this complication. In the mitral position, it has been the experience at Rabin Medical Center that Amplatzer plug III, implanted from a retrograde approach, has a particularly high rate of leaflet entrapment, as the disk at the tail of the device is thin and hinged.

The angulation of the leak and the valve ring also impacts on leaflet entrapment. In the mitral position, devices that are located in leaks that are perpendicular to the valve ring are less likely to catch on the leaflet compared to leaks that surround the edge of the ring so that the jet direction is almost parallel to the valve. In the aortic position, most leaks are from the aortic sinus, in parallel to the valve ring and remote from the moving leaflet, so that leaflet entrapment is rare.

Leaflet entrapment is easily recognized on fluoroscopy and echocardiography before release of the device. So in the majority of cases, this is not a complication but a finding that requires readjustment of the device's position and, if not successful, removal of the device and replacing it, either with a smaller one, a different device type, or a change of approach, usually from retrograde to antegrade. It is mandatory to perform fluoroscopy in the pivot view before releasing the device, even if valve performance on echocardiography remains good. If after several attempts all devices and approaches fail, procedure failure has to be declared.

Rarely, a device that seems to be well placed changes configuration after release, catching on the leaflet. This then becomes a true complication, as the device has to be snared and removed, risking device embolization, or the patient has to undergo urgent operation.

Case No. 4

An 82-year-old gentleman with para-aortic leak had a large Amplatzer plug II device in one of two para-aortic leaks (Fig. 11.5). Valve function was normal on ICE, and the device was released. Only after disconnecting the device it was realized that no fluoroscopic pivot view was performed. On pivot view it was apparent that the device limited the opening of one of the aortic valve disks. As the valve hemodynamics remained satisfactory, and retrieval of the device at this stage appeared to carry a significant risk of embolization, it was decided to leave it in place. After several weeks, having confirmed that valve function remained satisfactory, a second leak was closed, resulting in marked clinical improvement. This was a preventable complication, but luckily, on this rare occasion, having missed it before device release has proven beneficial to the patient.

11.6.2 Leaflet Erosion

Usually leaks around bioprosthetic valves are easier to close because there is no issue of leaflet entrapment. However, leaflet erosion by large devices has been described. This of course is a late complication that cannot be appreciated during the procedure [17].

11.6.3 Device Embolization

All kinds of plugs used for paravalvular leak closure are detachable, meaning their release is controlled by the operator. Usually the device is securely located inside the leak tunnel when the sheath is pulled backward and the release mechanism is exposed. Therefore, the risk of device embolization is low [1, 18]. Embolization may occur when a device has been released and a second one is placed next to it. Also, in cases where several devices are delivered simultaneously through a single sheath, the devices are exteriorized from the sheath in the ventricle or atrium and then pulled back into the tunnel leak. This increases the risk of inadvertent release of the device resulting in embolization. Rarely, the device can be separated from the delivery cable when still in the delivery sheath. At that stage, it can be reattached to the cable. The device should be pulled out and remounted properly on the cable before reintroduction. It is advisable to always pull on the cable during delivery of a device, before exteriorizing it. By just pushing all the way through, one may not be aware that the

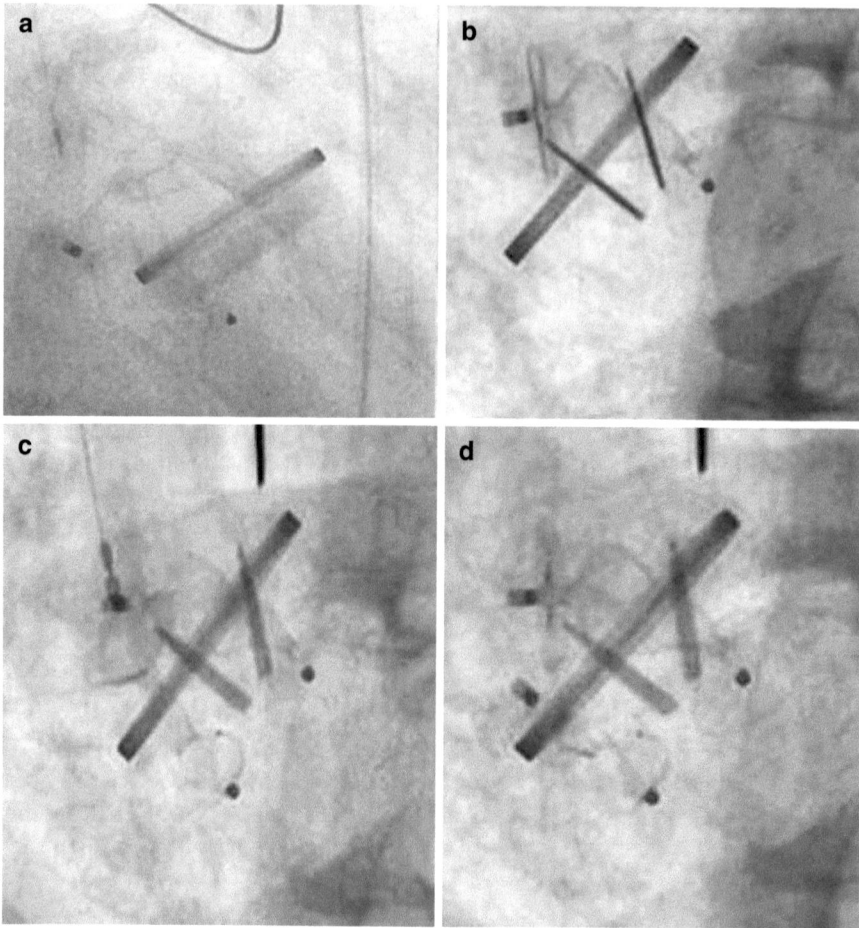

Fig. 11.5 Closure of paravalvular aortic leak with Amplatzer plug II. (**a**) Device released after confirming normal valve function on echocardiography but without confirming unobstructed leaflet motion on fluoroscopic pivot view. (**b**) Pivot view showing limitation of leaflet motion by the occluder. (**c**) As valve function remained satisfactory over time, a second device, Amplatzer plug III, was implanted in a second leak, this time with pivot view confirmed and (**d**) released

cable has detached. An embolized device can usually be retrieved percutaneously. If successful, the procedure can be continued. In the literature, only late embolization or inability to retrieve a device count as a procedural complication [7].

11.6.4 Late Dislodgement of Devices

Introducing metal mesh devices under pressure into the crescent-shaped leaks imposes sustained radial forces on the surrounding tissue. This is particularly true for older devices, e.g., the Amplatzer duct occluder (ADO) I or muscular VSD occluders, that have a round shape and are made of thicker and more robust metal wires, compared to the oval-shaped, thin wire devices, e.g., the Amplatzer plug III. Considering the fact that the leak occurred in the first place because of weakness of the tissues to which the valve ring has been sutured, this constant pressure may increase tissue trauma and result in gradual expansion of the leak, with reappearance of the leak which may have initially been sealed off effectively.

On rare occasions, the tear of tissues around the device results in the device becoming unstable, changing shape and position, and even embolizing [19].

Case No. 5

A 75-year-old gentleman with severe para-mitral leak and end-stage renal failure had a ADO I placed in the leak. At first, there was leaflet entrapment, and in order to free the disk, the device was further pulled into the leak tunnel so that even the retention disk was distorted. This maneuver seemed to do the job, with acceptable residual leak. However, over a few months' period, the leak reappeared and gradually became worse than the original one. On fluoroscopy the device has moved out of the tunnel to the left atrium, regaining its original shape. It was still attached to the valve ring with a small amount of tissue (Fig. 11.6). The patient who was very sick had an urgent operation which he did not survive.

11.7   Coronary Orifice Obstruction

A rare complication, described in a case report, is obstruction of the right coronary artery orifice by an occluder device 2 months after closure of a para-aortic leak [20].

11.8   New or Worsening Hemolysis

Intravascular mechanical hemolysis, resulting from friction of erythrocytes with the rough surface of the leak edges, is an important complication of paravalvular leaks. It is usually the clinical presentation of smaller leaks, while the larger ones cause mainly congestive heart failure. When introducing a closure device into the leak, partially closing it, we make it both smaller and rougher, due to the metal surface of the device, thus increasing the potential for new or worsening hemolysis. In the initial experience at Rabin Medical Center, using mainly Amplatzer duct occluders, which almost invariably left residual leaks due to their round shape inside an oblong tear, almost half of the patients had worsening hemolysis [21]. However, in a recent series, the incidence of new or worsening hemolysis is much lower, particularly if only severe hemolysis, requiring blood transfusion, is considered. This is probably because most procedures nowadays make use of devices that fit better to the shape of the tear or of several smaller devices that achieve a higher rate of sealing [5, 7].

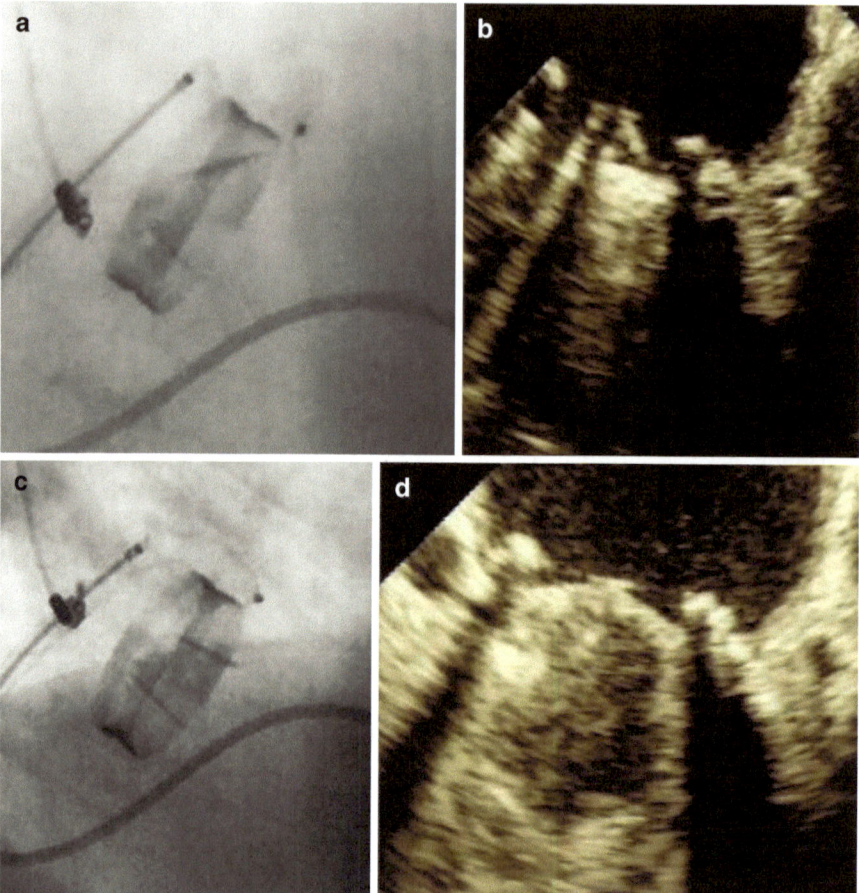

Fig. 11.6 (**a**) Fluoroscopic appearance of ADO I device impinging on valve leaflet. (**b**) TEE 2D frame showing the immobile leaflet. (**c**) Pulling back on the device, getting the retention disk in the PVL tunnel frees the valve leaflet. (**d**) Residual leak is acceptable and device is released (**e-f**). (**g**) On TEE several months later, regurgitation is severe. (**h**) Fluoroscopy shows the device has everted entirely into the left atrium, still hanging on the valve ring

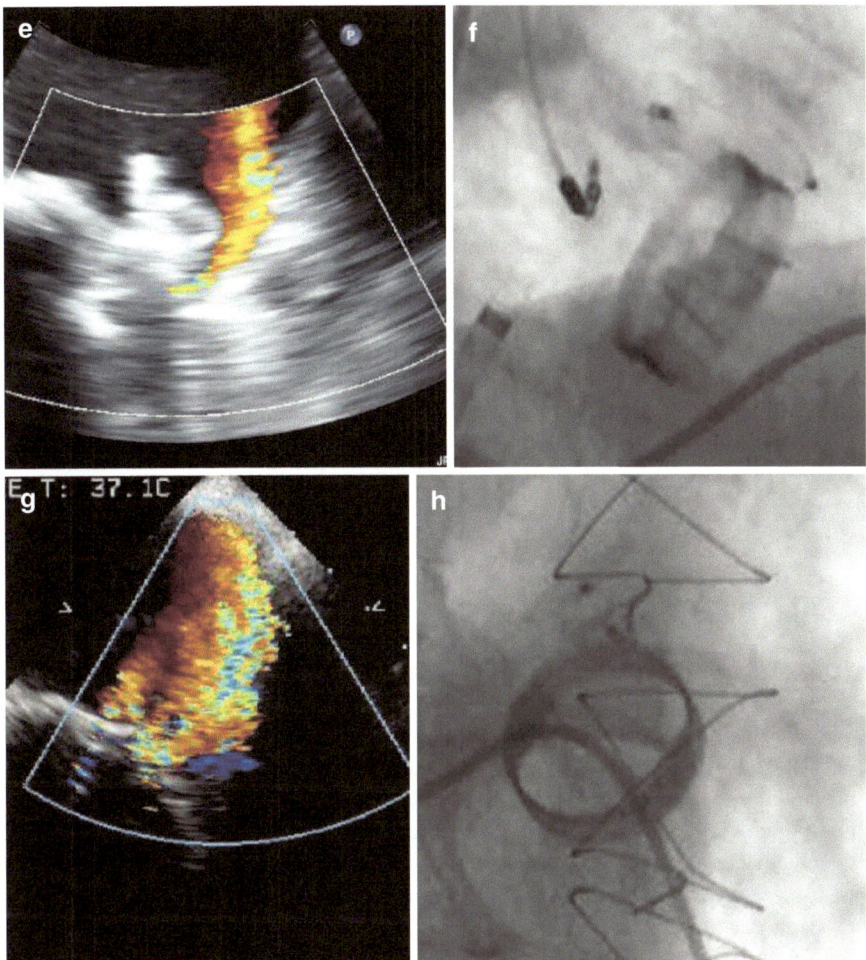

Fig. 11.6 (continued)

11.9 General Complications of Structural Interventions

Besides the above complications regarding the specifics of paravalvular leak closure, patients undergoing PVL closure can experience contrast media-related
nephropathy, stroke due to thromboembolism, infection including endocarditis [22],
and complications related to general anesthesia.

The patients treated for paravalvular leaks are often very sick with heart failure,
pulmonary hypertension, anemia, and arrhythmia. They are more likely to have
complications, and the impact of those complications may be more hazardous than
similar complications in younger and healthier subjects. However, they also carry a
very poor surgical risk.

Although head-to-head comparison of surgical and catheter-based interventions
for paravalvular leak closure has not been performed and will not likely take place
in the future, recent publications show a clear advantage of the percutaneous
approach to paravalvular leak closure compared to historical surgical series [1].

11.10 Procedure Failure as a "Complication"

Taking into consideration the advantages of the percutaneous techniques, procedure
failure, even if no complications had occurred, should be considered a worrying
event, as the patient will require reoperation with a higher morbidity and mortality.

Therefore, it is mandatory to undertake every possible effort in order for the
procedure to succeed. This involves careful planning, a large and varied arsenal of
equipment, flexibility of thought during the procedure, changing approaches where
deemed necessary, and the involvement of an experienced operator. Not less important is the quality of the supporting imaging team, in the planning and during the
procedure.

References

1. Cruz-Gonzalez I, Rama-Merchan JC, Calvert PA, Rodríguez-Collado J, Barreiro-Pérez M,
   Martín-Moreiras J, et al. Percutaneous closure of paravalvular leaks: a systematic review.
   J Interv Cardiol. 2016;29(4):382–92.
2. Taramasso M, Maisano F, Latib A, Denti P, Guidotti A, Sticchi A, et al. Conventional surgery and transcatheter closure via surgical transapical approach for paravalvular leak repair in
   high-risk patients: results from a single-centre experience. Eur Heart J Cardiovasc Imaging.
   2014;15(10):1161–7.
3. Sorajja P, Cabalka AK, Hagler DJ, Rihal CS. Long-term follow-up of percutaneous repair of
   paravalvular prosthetic regurgitation. J Am Coll Cardiol. 2011;58(21):2218–24.
4. Mookadam F, Raslan SF, Jiamsripong P, Jalal U, Murad MH. Percutaneous closure of
   mitral paravalvular leaks: a systematic review and meta-analysis. J Heart Valve Dis.
   2012;21(2):208–17.

5. Smolka G, Pysz P, Wojakowski W, Ochała A, Peszek-Przybyła E, Roleder T, et al. Clinical manifestations of heart failure abate with transcatheter aortic paravalvular leak closure using Amplatzer vascular plug II and III devices. J Invasive Cardiol. 2013;25(5):226–31.
6. Smolka G, Pysz P, Jasiński M, Roleder T, Peszek-Przybyła E, Ochała A, et al. Multiplug paravalvular leak closure using Amplatzer Vascular Plugs III: a prospective registry. Catheter Cardiovasc Interv. 2016;87(3):478–87.
7. Calvert PA, Northridge D, Malik IS, Shapiro L, Ludman P, Qureshi SA, et al. Percutaneous device closure of paravalvular leak: combined experience from the United Kingdom and Ireland. Circulation. 2016;134(13):934–44.
8. Wasmer K, Zellerhoff S, Köbe J, Mönnig G, Pott C, Dechering DG, et al. Incidence and management of inadvertent puncture and sheath placement in the aorta during attempted transseptal puncture. Europace. 2017;19(3):447–57.
9. Mijangos-Vázquez R, García-Montes JA, Zabal-Cerdeira C. Aortic iatrogenic perforation during transseptal puncture and successful occlusion with Amplatzer ductal occluder in a case of mitral paravalvular leak closure. Catheter Cardiovasc Interv. 2016;88(2):312–5.
10. Smolka G, Pysz P, Jasinski M, Gocoł R, Domaradzki W, Hudziak D, et al. Transapical closure of mitral paravalvular leaks with use of Amplatzer vascular plug III. J Invasive Cardiol. 2013;25(10):497–501.
11. Nijenhuis VJ, Swaans MJ, Post MC, Heijmen RH, de Kroon TL, Ten Berg JM. Open transapical approach to transcatheter paravalvular leakage closure: a preliminary experience. Circ Cardiovasc Interv. 2014;7(4):611–20.
12. Dudiy Y, Kliger C, Jelnin V, Elisabeth A, Kronzon I, Ruiz CE. Percutaneous transapical access: current status. EuroIntervention. 2014;10(Suppl U):U84–9.
13. Kappetein AP, Head SJ, Généreux P, Piazza N, van Mieghem NM, Blackstone EH, et al. Updated standardized endpoint definitions for transcatheter aortic valve implantation: the Valve Academic Research Consortium-2 consensus document (VARC-2). Eur J Cardiothorac Surg. 2012;42(5):S45–60.
14. Martinez CA, Cohen H, Ruiz CE. Wire entrapment through an aortic paravalvular leak. J Invasive Cardiol. 2010;22(7):E119–21.
15. Hein R, Wunderlich N, Robertson G, Wilson N, Sievert H. Catheter closure of paravalvular leak. EuroIntervention. 2006;2(3):318–25.
16. Nietlispach F, Johnson M, Moss RR, Wijesinghe N, Gurvitch R, Tay EL, et al. Transcatheter closure of paravalvular defects using a purpose-specific occluder. JACC Cardiovasc Interv. 2010;3(7):759–65.
17. Rogers JH, Morris AS, Takeda PA, Low RI. Bioprosthetic leaflet erosion after percutaneous mitral paravalvular leak closure. JACC Cardiovasc Interv. 2010;3(1):122–3.
18. Ruiz CE, Jelnin V, Kronzon I, Dudiy Y, Del Valle-Fernandez R, Einhorn BN, et al. Clinical outcomes in patients undergoing percutaneous closure of periprosthetic paravalvular leaks. J Am Coll Cardiol. 2011;58(21):2210–7.
19. Ussia GP, Scandura S, Calafiore AM, Mangiafico S, Meduri R, Galassi AR, et al. Images in cardiovascular medicine. Late device dislodgement after percutaneous closure of mitral prosthesis paravalvular leak with Amplatzer muscular ventricular septal defect occluder. Circulation. 2007;115(8):e208–10.
20. Hernández-Enríquez M, Ascaso M, Freixa X, Sandoval E, Giacchi G, Brugaletta S, et al. Late right coronary ostium occlusion after percutaneous aortic paravalvular leak closure: immediate results do not always predict long-term performance. J Invasive Cardiol. 2016;28(8):E69–70.
21. Shapira Y, Hirsch R, Kornowski R, Hasdai D, Assali A, Vaturi M, et al. Percutaneous closure of paravalvular leaks with Amplatzer occluders: feasibility, safety, and short term results. J Heart Valve Dis. 2007;16(3):305–13.
22. Lee CY, Ling FS, Knight PA. Endocarditis of Amplatzer occluder devices after percutaneous closure of a mitral paravalvular leak. Catheter Cardiovasc Interv. 2013;81(7):1249–52.

Chapter 12
Summary

Grzegorz Smolka, Wojciech Wojakowski, and Michał Tendera

12.1 General Perspective

The first papers pointing out to the potential use of transcatheter techniques to manage patients with paravalvular leaks (PVL) were published in 2011 [1–3].

As patients with PVL are generally at high surgical risk, this approach has rapidly gained considerable interest, as reflected by both the European and the US practice guidelines [4–6]. As soon as in 2012, the ESC Guidelines on the management of valvular heart disease included a statement that transcatheter closure of PVL is feasible but experience is limited, and there is presently no conclusive evidence to show a consistent efficiency. It was concluded that transcatheter PVL closure may be considered in selected patients in whom surgical reintervention is deemed high risk or is contraindicated [4], but there was no formal recommendation on the use of this approach. In the 2014 AHA/ACC Guidelines [5], the procedure was assigned class IIa, level of evidence B, accompanied by the following statement: "Percutaneous repair of paravalvular regurgitation is reasonable in patients with prosthetic heart valves and intractable hemolysis or NYHA class III/IV heart failure (HF) who are at high risk for surgery and have anatomic features suitable for catheter-based therapy when performed in centers with expertise in the procedure." The 2017 AHA/ACC Guideline update did not change the indications for the transcatheter PVL closure [6].

In principle, the official approach to the method on both sides of the Atlantic is similar and indicates that the transcatheter PVL treatment is potentially beneficial, but needs further research to define its optimal place in the management of patients with PVL.

G. Smolka (✉) • W. Wojakowski • M. Tendera
Department of Cardiology and Structural Heart Diseases, School of Medicine in Katowice, Medical University of Silesia, Katowice, Poland
e-mail: gsmolka@me.com

© Springer Nature Singapore Pte Ltd. 2017   179
G. Smolka et al. (eds.), *Transcatheter Paravalvular Leak Closure*,
DOI 10.1007/978-981-10-5400-6_12

12.2   Limitations of Available Data

Transcatheter PVL closure is technically demanding, as morphology of the defects represents great diversity and may be extremely complex. For that reason, imaging techniques, delivery systems, and choice of the occluders are still challenging. Over the last years, a substantial progress has occurred, which is apparent in such areas as 3D echo navigation [7, 8] or fusion imaging available at the time of intervention [9]. This prompted a widespread interest in transcatheter PVL closure using both transvascular (arterial or venous) and transapical (hybrid) approach. Importantly, national registries, as well as a meta-analysis of the available data, suggested that transcatheter PVL treatment may result in clinical improvement [10–13].

It needs to be stressed that the criteria used to define a therapeutic success have not been well established. Both technical and clinical success are not easy to define. Successful occluder deployment alone is not sufficient, since even with multiple devices a residual leak may still be present. Clinically, the difficulty is well illustrated by the fact that a technically successful procedure may be associated with both an improvement and a deterioration of hemolytic anemia [14, 15]. Hence, a quest has been made for standardization of clinical endpoints after the PVL closure [16].

Most importantly, however, there are no randomized comparisons of transcatheter with surgical PVL treatment. Moreover, with some exceptions, such comparisons are unlikely to be undertaken in the future. This is due to the fact that several patient groups, such as those with infectious endocarditis, valvular prosthesis instability, or the need for concomitant CABG, do not qualify for transcatheter PVL closure. In addition, there is an intermediate group of patients who are not optimal candidates for transcatheter repair, but may be considered for it, e.g., those with multiple small leaks involving a large part of the prosthetic ring. Recent data, however, point out to the fact that surgical approach is connected with considerably higher risk than the percutaneous treatment, even when corrected for the known confounders [17]. Thus, randomized comparisons of the two approaches may be deemed impractical or even unethical. Still, comparison of the outcome in patients qualifying for transcatheter treatment with surgical approach on one side, and with medical treatment on the other side, can represent appropriate models to be tested in randomized studies.

12.3   Future Directions

Future directions in the development of transcatheter PVL closure should be focused on technical and clinical aspects of the procedure.

On the technical side, there is a need for refinement of the imaging methods and development of dedicated occluders and delivery systems. Undoubtedly, refinement of fusion imaging, involving the 3D echo, CT and fluoroscopy, and possibly also devoted sizing balloon techniques, is necessary to better establish the indications, facilitate the procedure, and objectively assess its outcome. Thus far, different types of occluders have been utilized for PVL closure. The AVP II and III occluders (Amplatzer vascular plug II and III, Abbott) have been most commonly used. Although sometimes the AVP III occlude is addressed as PVL dedicated [18], it has not been formally registered for this indication. On the other hand, the PLD occluder (paravalvular leak device, Occlutech) does have the CE mark, but is not registered in the USA. The data on its application in clinical practice are so far limited [19, 20].

Importantly, occluder delivery systems are suboptimal. A dedicated, steerable system could dramatically facilitate the procedure, especially in case of paramitral leaks.

Ongoing studies, including the "Integrated system for trascatheter closure of paravalvular leaks (VALE)" (STRATEGMED2/269488/7/NCBR/2015), are likely to contribute to the improvement of imaging techniques, as well as to the development of dedicated occluders and delivery systems for the transcatheter PVL closure.

Recent publication of the Paravalvular Leak Academic Research Consortium, proposing criteria of PVL grading, proper imaging, and outcome measures [21], is of paramount importance for the development of the method. This is a state-of-the-art document, standardizing definitions and outcome measures for future research.

It is likely that the current, restricted indications for the transcatheter PVL closure will be broadened in the future. Our data indicate that in patients with para-aortic leaks, early intervention may result in the regression of left ventricular end-diastolic volume, which, in conjunction with a low periprocedural mortality, may favor an earlier timing of the procedure [12]. In case of mitral PVL the situation is more complex. The improvement in left ventricular volumes and ejection fraction has not been proven, but there is a consistent improvement in the NYHA class [22].

12.4 Conclusions

Transcatheter PVL closure is a promising and rapidly evolving field. Availability of globally acceptable definitions and research goals should prompt international collaboration on this clinically and scientifically important topic.

References

1. Ruiz CE, Jelnin V, Kronzon I, et al. Clinical outcomes in patients undergoing percutaneous closure of periprosthetic paravalvular leaks. J Am Coll Cardiol. 2011;58:2210–7.
2. Sorajja P, Cabalka AK, Hagler DJ, Rihal CS. Long-term follow-up of percutaneous repair of paravalvular prosthetic regurgitation. J Am Coll Cardiol. 2011;58:2218–24.

3. Sorajja P, Cabalka AK, Hagler DJ, Rihal CS. Percutaneous repair of paravalvular prosthetic regurgitation: acute and 30-day outcomes in 115 patients. Circ Cardiovasc Interv. 2011;4:314–21.
4. Vahanian A, Alfieri O, Andreotti F, et al. Guidelines on the Management of Valvular Heart Disease (version 2012): the Joint Task Force on the Management of Valvular Heart Disease of the European Society of Cardiology (ESC) and the European Association for Cardio-Thoracic Surgery (EACTS). Eur J Cardiothorac Surg. 2012;42:S1–44.
5. Nishimura RA, Otto CM, Bonow RO, et al. 2014 AHA/ACC guideline for the management of patients with valvular heart disease: executive summary: a report of the American College of Cardiology/American Heart Association Task Force on practice guidelines. J Am Coll Cardiol. 2014;63:2438–88.
6. Nishimura RA, Otto CM, Bonow RO et al. 2017 AHA/ACC focused update of the 2014 AHA/ACC guideline for the Management of Patients with Valvular Heart Disease: a report of the American College of Cardiology/American Heart Association Task Force on clinical practice guidelines. J Am Coll Cardiol. 2017.
7. Rodriguez Munoz D, Lazaro Rivera C, Zamorano Gomez JL. Guidance of treatment of perivalvular prosthetic leaks. Curr Cardiol Rep. 2014;16:430.
8. Arribas-Jimenez A, Rama-Merchan JC, Barreiro-Perez M, et al. Utility of real-time 3-dimensional transesophageal echocardiography in the assessment of mitral paravalvular leak. Circ J. 2016;80:738–44.
9. Kliger C, Jelnin V, Sharma S, et al. CT angiography-fluoroscopy fusion imaging for percutaneous transapical access. JACC Cardiovasc Imaging. 2014;7:169–77.
10. Calvert PA, Northridge DB, Malik IS, et al. Percutaneous device closure of paravalvular leak: combined experience from the United Kingdom and Ireland. Circulation. 2016;134:934–44.
11. Millan X, Skaf S, Joseph L, et al. Transcatheter reduction of paravalvular leaks: a systematic review and meta-analysis. Can J Cardiol. 2015;31:260–9.
12. Smolka G, Pysz P, Wojakowski W, et al. Clinical manifestations of heart failure abate with transcatheter aortic paravalvular leak closure using Amplatzer vascular plug II and III devices. J Invasive Cardiol. 2013;25:226–31.
13. Garcia E, Arzamendi D, Jimenez-Quevedo P, et al. Outcomes and predictors of success and complications for paravalvular leak closure: an analysis of the SpanisH real-wOrld paravalvular LEaks closure (HOLE) registry. EuroIntervention. 2017;12(16):1962–8.
14. Smolka G, Pysz P, Ochala A, et al. Transcatheter paravalvular leak closure and hemolysis—a prospective registry. Arch Med Sci. 2017;13:575–84.
15. De Bruyn A, Dendale P, Benit E. Hemolysis after percutaneous paravalvular leak repair. Acta Clin Belg. 2016:1–3.
16. Ruiz CE, Mathur AP. Paravalvular leak closure: time to standardize clinical endpoints? JACC Cardiovasc Interv. 2016;9:2427–8.
17. Angulo-Llanos R, Sarnago-Cebada F, Rivera AR, et al. Two-year follow up after surgical versus percutaneous paravalvular leak closure: a non-randomized analysis. Catheter Cardiovasc Interv. 2016;88:626–34.
18. Nietlispach F, Johnson M, Moss RR, et al. Transcatheter closure of paravalvular defects using a purpose-specific occluder. JACC Cardiovasc Interv. 2010;3:759–65.
19. Smolka G, Pysz P, Kozlowski M, et al. Transcatheter closure of paravalvular leaks using a paravalvular leak device—a prospective polish registry. Postepy Kardiol Interwencyjnej. 2016;12:128–34.
20. Goktekin O, Vatankulu MA, Ozhan H, et al. Early experience of percutaneous paravalvular leak closure using a novel Occlutech occluder. EuroIntervention. 2016;11:1195–200.
21. Ruiz CE, Hahn RT, Berrebi A et al. Clinical trial principles and endpoint definitions for paravalvular leaks in surgical prosthesis: an expert statement. Eur Heart J. 2017.
22. Smolka G, Pysz P, Jasinski M, et al. Transapical closure of mitral paravalvular leaks with use of amplatzer vascular plug III. J Invasive Cardiol. 2013;25:497–501.